GARLAND STUDIES ON

# THE ELDERLY IN AMERICA

*A collection of monographs and dissertations addressing specific problems facing the elderly in a changing America*

EDITED BY
**STUART BRUCHEY**
Columbia University

A Garland Series

# RETIREMENT AND MEN'S PHYSICAL AND MENTAL HEALTH

Raoul Louis Betancourt

**GARLAND PUBLISHING**
*New York & London*
*1991*

**Library of Congress Cataloging-in-Publication Data**


Betancourt, Raoul Louis.
    Retirement and men's physical and mental health / Raoul Louis Betancourt.
        p.   cm. — (Garland studies on the elderly in America)
    Includes bibliographical references.
    ISBN 0-8153-0508-7
    1. Men—Retirement—Health aspects. 2. Men—Health and hygiene. 3. Men—
    Mental health.
    I. Title. II. Series.
    RA564.83.B48 1991
    613'.04234—dc20

91-37219
CIP

**Printed on acid-free 250-year-life paper**

**MANUFACTURED IN THE UNITED STATES OF AMERICA**

To mother and grandmother whose love and confidence are strength and inspiration, and to the memories of my grandfather and great-grandparents whose marks remain forever in my life.

# ACKNOWLEDGEMENTS

I extend sincerest gratitude to my dissertation committee at the University of Michigan in 1989: Dr. Joseph Veroff, Dr. Ruth Dunkle, Dr. Charles Garvin and Dr. John Hagen. I am also thankful to Dr. Toni Antonucci and Dr. James Jackson at the Institute for Social Research, University of Michigan.

# TABLE OF CONTENTS

# LIST OF FIGURES

# LIST OF TABLES

# LIST OF APPENDICES

# Chapter I

# RETIREMENT AS A MAJOR LIFE EVENT

Retirement is an experience that nearly all older men experience. The number of retired men is currently increasing because the population of all older adults is expanding very rapidly. Therefore, older men's retirement has become an especially significant social issue—an issue that is frequently accompanied by physical and mental health problems.

The literature has been inconclusive regarding beneficial and harmful effects of retirement upon the physical and mental well-being of older men. However, the main hypothesis of this work is that retirement is a *harmful* experience for the physical and mental health of older men. The secondary hypothesis states that when retired men also suffer death of a spouse or significant other, their physical and mental health become worse. An examination of these hypotheses composes the bulk of this study. A social problem that concerns retired men is discussed in the final chapter of this study: What happens when older retired men in America are faced with health problems and must deal with an unsatisfactory health care system.

This dissertation will begin by reviewing relevant social science literature concerning the retirement of older men with several objectives. First, the importance of worklife to men in America is discussed, and this serves to preface a description of retirement as a major social loss for older men. Second, demographic trends related to retirement are pointed out. Third, a brief history of retirement policy is given, followed by a discussion of the reasons for retirement. Fourth, the impact of men's personal resources on coping with retirement is examined. Fifth, the disruptive effect of retirement on older men's social situation is discussed, comprising a large section of the chapter. This section is followed by an examination of retirement as a source of stress. The chapter concludes with an account of the general negative effect of retirement on retirees' financial resources.

## How Retirement Affects Male Workers

In our labor-intensive and consumer-oriented society, the private enterprise system sets "work" as the one route American men must follow to become successful. Success is generally equated with purchasing power for material possessions. However, men do not work *only* to provide themselves and their families with material goods; men find that work is also an activity that offers social and psychological benefits such as peer support, socialization opportunities, and self-esteem boosters.

The work role generally benefits a worker's well-being. The worker's job represents an opportunity for positive accomplishment and increases self-esteem. The job also allows outlets for social participation and stimulates the development of other social roles (Mutran and Reitzes, 1981). MacBride (1976) emphasizes the important role of worklife to the worker by stating that Freud describes work as securely attaching man to a part of reality—to the human community. Thus, most men become physically and mentally involved in their job environment and identify themselves as achieving some level of success in American society (Kremer, 1985). The daily structuring of time and activities in the workplace permits realization of these above-mentioned social commodities (Robinson et al., 1985). Many working men may thus find life as a whole to be extremely satisfying when they find their work life to be self-affirming. However, most men must eventually relinquish this often beneficial worker role when they retire.

It is difficult to define retirement precisely. However, there are some elements common to most retirement experiences (Atchley, 1976). For instance, men usually retire when they are fifty years old or older and, as a general rule, stop working completely or only then work part-time. Most older men also give up most or all of their work-related personal contacts. In effect, they lose much of their peer support and primary set of social ties. Retirement often acts to disrupt seriously older men's social situation for the remainder of their lives (Atchley, 1976).

Retirement can encompass different individual experiences for men nearing retirement age. One reason for this is that retirement experiences are influenced primarily by the worker's former job (Bortz, 1972). Thus, retirement can be as diverse as the many different types of work settings. For example, blue-collar workers view retirement as a different sort of life event than do white-collar workers. Moreover, retirement's effects in general may be unanticipated and thus harmful (Palmore, 1964; Parnes and Nestel, 1981; Bradford, 1979). Consequently, older men often experience retirement as an overwhelmingly stressful life event.

To reinforce the importance of retirement as a major event in men's lives, Atchley (1976) designs a theoretical framework concerned with a specific enumeration of the stages of retirement. First, he theoretically links the retirement process to the context of changing social environments of aging persons by carefully integrating the retirement process into the more encompassing human aging process. He then illustrates retirement to be a stressful life event that is heavily affected by changes in the retiree's social environment and health status. The social environment is constantly changing according to Atchley. These changes usually affect each individual's health and social situations that, in turn, affect the retirement experience. For instance, an older worker may suddenly lose his spouse through death. His private social system outside of work, as a result, is suddenly and markedly altered. This change may negatively affect his physical and mental health, and the remainder of his retired life.

Atchley characterizes the retirement experience as integrally temporal (Haynes et al., 1977). The stages of the process are:

**Pre-retirement:** There is little dread of retirement here. Retirees have fantasies of what retired life will be like; then as the time becomes close at hand they feel growing negativity.

**Honeymoon:** Retirees now experience the novelty of freedom and leisure (a function of physical health and resources).

**Disenchantment:** In this phase, reality sets in. There are feelings of let-down and, perhaps, poor physical health.

**Reorientation:** Now, there is not much "honeymoon" to enjoy.

**Stability:** Retired life becomes routine and functional. Physical and mental health change because of the aging process.

**Termination:** This is the final stage of illness and/or death.

In this concise way, Atchley relates retirement experiences to the larger social environment, and he accounts for the retired person's often negative physical and mental health changes.

## Demographic Trends Affecting Retirement

Retirement issues obviously become more important as elderly populations increase. Adults in America who are 65 years old and over have been growing more numerous since World War II. However, only in the past 25 years has this population growth become a recognized national issue that encompasses labor, retirement, and health concerns (Palmore, 1964; Morrison, 1983; Robinson et al., 1985). Morrison says this general growth trend of older adults is more evident today than 45 years ago because of unanticipated changes in fertility rates from the late 1940s until the 1960s.

While the birth rate in America increased steadily from 1945 to 1960, it began to level off shortly after 1960 and declined markedly until 1970 (Morrison, 1983). These population shifts affected the demographic make-up of the American people in two important ways. First, the proportion of the total population that persons aged 65 and over represent steadily increased, as the following data illustrate. In *1950*, the group 65 years and older was 8.1 percent of the total population; in *1980*, it was 11.2 percent of the total population; and in *2030*, its projected figure is 18.3 percent of the total population (Russell, 1981). These population shifts mean that along with an increasing older population, American society will also have more people who are retired. Second, there is a decline in the young adult (22-30 years) proportion of the population. This population decline, in juxtaposition to the earlier mentioned population increase, acts to emphasize the already growing older population.

Moreover, there has been uneven growth across subgroups of adults over 55 year of age. In 1982, adults 55 to 64 years of age comprised 9.5 percent of the population. By 2030, they are expected to increase slightly and make up 10.4 percent of the total population. In 1982, adults 65 to 74 years of age comprised 6.7 percent of the population. By 2030, they should increase moderately and make up 10.2 percent of the population. Lastly, in 1982, adults 75 years and older represented 4.4 percent of the population. By 2030, they should almost double and account for 7.9 percent of the total population in America (Morrison, 1983).

Of this last group, the proportion of adults *85 years of age and older* is growing at a faster rate than any other segment of the older population, as well as any segment of the general population (Russell, 1981). This growth is important to society because increasing age is positively correlated with declining health (Minkler, 1981b). Consequently, the aging of the population is becoming a more complex social reality for two reasons: 1) the dramatic increase in the number of older Americans, and 2) the failure of American society to plan effectively to solve the social and health problems that result from this growth. This population growth challenges health policies in America designed for smaller older populations, and strains the limited resources of current programs designed for older adults (Morrison 1988).

Other demographic factors such as marital status, income levels, and educational achievement also influence retirement. These factors may determine differing retirement experiences among older men and the variety of consequent needs (Parnes and Nestel, 1981; Palmore, 1964). Palmore states that economic factors strongly influence retirement, and that low-income males are *more* likely to retire despite fewer material resources than middle and higher income individuals. Low-income males view retirement as a clear relief to their working lives despite the income loss. This factor contributes to the poverty and near-poverty rates common among a significant portion of retired older men.

Educational attainment particularly influences certain men's decision to retire. In fact, research has shown that education affects retirement more strongly than income (Durbin et al., 1984). For instance, college-educated men are likely to plan for *early* retirement, despite the fact that many of these men earn high incomes. The desire of these men to change their social situation is the stimulus to retire.

## History of Retirement Policy

Mandatory retirement and the Social Security Program were adopted in American society in the 1930s primarily as economic measures (Morrison, 1983). Policy-makers saw these programs as socially acceptable means of reducing the labor force during the economically-spare times of the depression years when employers wanted younger, cheaper, and more productive labor. Moreover, these programs were politically motivated because of the federal goal to institute programs that added popular support to the current administration. Humanitarian concern for the lives of older Americans did *not* influence this program development (Minkler, 1981b).  With such unprecedented and attractive economic motives for both employers and workers, however, many people were forced to retire while others decided to retire at 65 years of age or earlier.

Today, this pattern continues.  Despite recent federal legislation that extends the mandatory retirement age from 65 to 70, the rate of retirement has not decreased (Parnes and Nestel, 1981; Morrison, 1988).  Although many workers today are no longer being *forced* to retire at age 65, *voluntary* retirement among white collar professional Caucasian males aged 58-69 years remains common.  It is ironic that many of these white collar men are still relatively healthy and not facing mandatory retirement (Gustman and Steinmeier, 1984).

## Reasons for Retirement

As mentioned earlier, demographic factors can *influence* the type of retirement experience men have and contribute to the quality of the experience.  Likewise, a major *reason* for retirement is demographic.  Poor physical health causes retirement among large numbers of low-income blue-collar workers of different racial and ethnic backgrounds (Eisdorfer, 1972).  In research on middle-aged, blue-collar male workers who had coronary by-pass surgery, Love (1980) determines that there are three other factors in these men's lives that interact with poor physical health to predict retirement after this mid-life surgery.  They are: 1) having an unemployment period before the surgery, 2) having a physically strenuous job, and 3) having low educational attainment.

These numerous factors influence the route and timing of a man's retirement and give the experience unique characteristics (Minkler, 1981b).  However, they are not the only influential factors.  Some men retire because they desire a new social situation for old age.  For example, men can withdraw from their occupations voluntarily to enjoy more leisure time (Atchley, 1982).  Other men do not have such options because the basis of retirement is built into their employment policy.  As Durbin et al. (1984) state, these men leave the job "passively" without much sense of control because of mandatory retirement.  Hence, the retirement decision can be *influenced* by objective conditions like physical health, income, education and employment policy, and subjective conditions like mental health conditions (Lazarus and DeLongis, 1983).

## Impact of Personal Resources on
## Coping with Retirement

Retirement literature describes the retirement experience as one that makes "new and unfamiliar" demands upon the lives of retirees (Cassel, 1976b). Certain characteristics of the retirement situation may indeed be "unfamiliar." For instance, men may not be able to cope in their retired lives because they never developed the necessary skills. This is especially true because retirement highlights some unresolved incongruities from earlier in life in the relationship between male retirees and their social systems (Cassel, 1976b; Minkler, 1981b).

For instance, environmental demands that accompany retirement require men to use effective coping strategies to prevent retired life from becoming unmanageably stressful. Some retired men find retirement's demands to be overwhelming because as younger men they did not develop adequate coping skills to deal with stressful situations (Parnes and Nestel, 1984). Therefore, as older men they may find themselves helpless in the face of stress, may *reject* their past lives, and may develop attitudes of despair (Keith, 1985).

However, other older men cope with retirement by *not rejecting* their past lives but struggling instead to *prevent* the loss of all of their life's "commitment" (Ryff, 1985). "'Commitment' is defined as the sharing of knowledge and skill, and the assumption of leadership and decision-making roles for other people." These retirees do not reject life's commitment and "disengage"; rather, they continue to "engage" themselves with new activities and discover new purposes in life (Goudy and Reger, 1985).

In a similar vein, Maddox (1970) employs a life-span perspective using a framework based on the work of Erik Erikson. Maddox emphasizes that the effects of retirement are a function of men's personal biography and the details of their adult psychological development. Similarly, Nadelson (1969) writes that older men cope with new events by utilizing all they have inherited and learned in past life stages. Having coped successfully in previous stages does not guarantee one will succeed in present or future stages, but it is a necessary prerequisite.

Thus, post-retirement coping behaviors are difficult to predict because pre-retirement *attitudes* are not easy to categorize reliably in a psychological scale. Attitudes toward retirement represent men's psychological assessment of what they imagine retirement will be like. Older men develop different attitudes toward retirement because adult worklife is terribly diverse in American society. While men work, their individual mental health, the availability of retirement benefits, and uncertain economic conditions have strong effects upon their ability to conceptualize their future lives as retirees (Rakowski, 1979; Lazarus and DeLongis, 1983; Morrison, 1983). The degree to which older workers can conceptualize retirement as a positive experience influences their ability to subsequently cope with that experience.

It follows that relationships between pre-retirement *attitudes* and post-retirement *behaviors* do exist. For example, Keith (1985) finds that men's pre-retirement attitudes are significantly related to post-retirement coping difficulties. Palmore (1976) finds that negative pre-retirement attitudes are related to retirement adjustment difficulties and also correlate with retirees' low activity level (their poor use of leisure time).

However, as men age and approach retirement, they may not be able to fulfill these psychological expectations because their personal resources are no longer sufficient to make their new retired life satisfactory. Inaccurate and sluggish perceptions, failing memory, and poor reasoning contribute to this inability to cope with retirement (Birren, 1976; Minkler, 1981b).

Hansson (1986) and Cassel (1976b) see the same relationships and offer techniques to assist working men nearing retirement. Hansson suggests that men's pre-retirement attitudes can be positively geared to the future reality of the retirement event by pre-retirement training. To be successful, pre-retirement training must prepare workers to be able to handle the *major* psychological expectations that retirement brings along with it. These expectations include the ability of retirees to handle changes in their social environment, to manage aggression, and to accept the self and one's past life (Nadelson, 1969; Wolfe and Wolfe, 1975).

In general, pre-retirement training should make coping with retirement easier. A major reason for this positive result is that the retiree's self-esteem is maintained or boosted. Cassel says adequate preparedness for the demands of this "new and unfamiliar" retirement situation is an important factor for good mental health.

## Impact of Retirement on
## Older Men's Social Situation

## Social Networks and Social Support

Social networks in a person's life can often act as social *support* that reduces the stress of a life event such as retirement. This social support represents what other people *do* to help a person cope (Thoits, 1986). However, it is hard to divorce the social support a person receives from the coping resources a person has. The actual coping *process* actually might have begun sometime earlier in the stressed person's life. Thoits says a person first begins to cope when he forms appropriate social ties and networks in his life that may later act as social support in a time of environmental demands. For example, social support can frequently be useful to an individual when the support is in the form of instrumental or material aid given in the time of need. This support can take the form of money, food, clothing, housing, or transportation.

The provision of meaningful *emotional* social support is a more complex matter, however. For effective emotional support, the social support systems in older men's lives must be characterized by a variety of social ties, frequent contacts, and important *meanings* assigned to the relationships (Coyne and DeLongis, 1986; Heller et al., 1986; Lieberman, 1986). Some researchers have suggested that the "perceived" rather than the "actual" social support received is more influential for good mental health (Heller et al., 1986). They define "perceived" social support as the appraisals made by a man of his own social support system that enhances his own self-esteem. He may not need actual support at the time of the appraisal, but he is self-assured and satisfied with the likelihood of receiving it. Thus, his satisfaction with perceived or actual support, rather than number of encounters, is a better gauge of support effectiveness.

Dependable social support can thus help older men to shape the meaning of retirement (Caspi and Elder, 1986). As older men retire, or approach retirement, efforts can be made to mobilize social support in their lives. Research with general adult populations has shown social support enhances retired life (Lieberman, 1986).

As mentioned in the beginning of this chapter, work provides men with opportunities for social outlets by systemically offering routine peer participation in the employment setting. Frequently, this work-related social system extends beyond work and overlaps with other personal or social activities. These types of social system activities contribute to the overall well-being of male workers.

In addition, social-support literature emphasizes that family and friends, as non-employment sources of social support, are among the most important social networks in assisting older men to cope with the stress of retirement (Kessler, 1982; Coyne and DeLongis, 1986). Research substantiates that older men frequently depend on spouses for satisfactory social support (Sussman, 1976). Other studies look at significant others per se, that is, family members other than a spouse, or friends (Gurin et al., 1960; Roberto and Scott, 1986; Thoits, 1986; Wethington and Kessler, 1986).

Satisfactory social support positively influences the mental health of adults. Gurin et al. find that in a sample of adults, marital satisfaction increases as older adults age. Spouses usually have provided various important forms of support to each other throughout their married life, and they depend upon that support for their well-being. If a spouse suddenly dies, the survivor's mental health can be severely damaged.

A "significant other" can also assume the role of providing social support and social satisfaction. Thoits (1986) discusses how significant others can assist distressed individuals to change the meanings of stressful situations and, if necessary, to change their reactions to these situations. Significant others are perceived by the survivor to be available in times of need, and consequently, these relationships have positive meaning to him. Thus, significant others conceivably can help older men deal with recent retirement (or the loss of a spouse) and help increase or maintain their feelings of life satisfaction.

Research has shown that those older men who have constructive coping skills also tend to have an effective social support network and good physical and mental health (Preston and Mansfield, 1984; Checkoway, 1988; Israel, 1988; Minkler, 1988; Cutrona et al., 1986). Unfortunately, though, research has also found that many older men fail to develop necessary coping skills to protect themselves against the stress of personal losses. For instance, many older men typically do not establish strong social relationships in their lives apart from their job except that of a spouse or close family members (Antonucci, 1983). In addition, Hansson (1986) finds that retirement does upset retirees' social systems and often results in the shrinking of men's support network, if they have one. When the social support network shrinks too much, men can find themselves socially isolated.

If retired men do not successfully establish personal and supportive ties in other social networks, and meet the demands of their changing social environment, they probably find retired life disturbing and unsatisfactory (Ingersoll, 1982). In many instances, older males who have lost spouses through death are in danger of becoming socially isolated because their spouses acted as the main providers of non-employment social support. The *loss* of a spouse or a significant other can be emotionally-damaging to some older men who may then become suicidal. Levitt et al., (1982) point out that men who *retire* and lose employment-related support, and experience the *death of a spouse/significant other* often develop extremely poor mental health and tend to be more suicidal than other groups of males.

## Role Shifts

It is harsh reality that most older men must shift from the work role to the retired role at least once in their lives. Societal pressures and expectations frequently cause  aging adult men to experience tensions in their lives as they attempt to fulfill the social role of retirement. For instance, the "larger society" in America (1) sanctions traditional marriages and family bonds to the exclusion of other important non-family relationships such as adult friendships, and (2) *does not* encourage men to develop a diverse system of social support to assist them in stressful role shifts. Moreover, American society values youth and productivity; aging and retirement are anathema to these values.

Older men who have recently retired must face two major role shifts. First, they must shift from their accustomed role of several decades as a member of the work force to the retired role. Second, they find themselves making this shift as *older* men in America. Older retired men may respond negatively to their new life circumstances because they find themselves in new roles that are stressful and uncomfortable. The base for their identities has shifted dramatically and they are ambivalent about future security.

## Retirement as a Source of Stress

The literature, therefore, asserts that retirement for older men severely may be stressful and upset their social situations (Holmes and Rahe, 1967; Cutrona et al., 1986; Cassel, 1976a; Cassel, 1976b; Lin et al., 1979; Linn, 1986; Preston and Mansfield, 1984). However, social scientists disagree on the origin of stress (Sells, 1970). Selye (1974) defines stress as a non-specific response of the body to *any* demand, regardless of whether the demand is pleasant or unpleasant. Elwell and Maltbie-Crannell (1981) define stress as an imbalance between the self-perceived demand placed on an individual and the self-perceived capability of responding to it. They theorize that the individual's social environment is where the self-perceived stressful demand manifests itself.

However, interactionist stress theoreticians such as Sells (1970) conceptualize *one* description of stress that is both externally *and* internally produced. In the case of retirement, stressful reactions are seen to flow from both internal sources (men's aging processes) and external sources (retirement upsetting men's social environment). Stress exists within man's self-perception and social context.

Stress levels vary among men according to their degree of involvement in life experiences or life events (Sells, 1970). Life experiences like work and retirement are closely related because each experience contributes to feelings of self-efficacy and self-esteem. Each of these experiences entails major personal involvement. More personal involvement in the experience intensifies the human response to stress whether the response is physical or psychological. Stress-responses occur because the life event possesses one of two characteristics according to Adam (1980): (1) *surprise* (as in retirement for poor health or death of a spouse or significant other that did not permit much preparation), (2) *a planned transition of major consequence* (such as "normal" retirement that may still be upsetting to men's lives).

Retirement may also trigger stress-responses because men often perceive themselves to be unable to meet the psychological demands of the event (Bradford, 1979; Palmore et al., 1979). These demands are related to men's self-perceptions of retirement and their self-esteem levels. The actual retirement experiences may not be similar to what was imagined or expected. Understandably, then, some researchers view retirement as highly stressful (Palmore et al., 1979; Bradford, 1979).

Such stress is even more likely to develop when life events are characterized by a conspicuous absence of important psychosocial elements such as "personal control" and "social support." Research documents that stress appears in environments where men have no personal control, as with mandatory retirement or the death of a spouse/significant other (Adam, 1980; Minkler, 1981a). Cassel (1976a) claims that this lack of control is common in men who are "marginal," that is, men who live on society's periphery and frequently have little meaningful social contact. Retirement's stress levels, thus, are seen as having particularly negative effects on factors such as men's self-esteem, life satisfaction, and satisfaction with health (Schnore, 1981; Eisdorfer, 1972; Nadelson, 1969; Quinn, 1981).

## Impact of Retirement on Financial Resources

Retirement may contribute to older men's poor mental health because retirement may reduce financial resources (Lazarus and DeLongis, 1983). While working, retired men may have been the only "breadwinner" in their households. Now as retirees, they are no longer the breadwinner. These older men must live with reduced incomes while also receiving government supplements like social security. Their spouses may receive some social security income as well. However, the financial resources in retired men's families are usually substantially reduced. Consequently, a transitional event like retirement causes men hardships in fulfilling basic and important life needs like food and shelter while it also weakens their self-esteem.

Many men lose the dollar-amount of their working salary when they retire, yet often this loss is somewhat compensated by a pension (Palmore et al., 1985). Pensions can pay up to 50 percent of the final salary or more, but pensions are not common, especially for blue-collar workers. Financial alternatives exist that attempt to offset salary loss and the lack of a pension. They are personal savings and federal subsidies.

In theory, retired men can depend upon accumulated lifetime personal savings to support them in retirement years. However, in reality, accumulated savings are not options for the majority of retired men. Many middle-class persons and nearly all lower-class persons cannot depend upon personal savings alone. Generally, only those persons who had substantial incomes while working can rely upon personal resources like trust funds, investments, and other assets to ensure a financially-secure retired life. Many retirees in America must depend upon Federal subsidies in the hopes of meeting the real and potential costs of old age (Russell, 1981).

Federal subsidies for retirees are of three types: work-related, age-related, and means-tested (Parnes and Nestel, 1981). As a work-related contributory Federal program, Social Security provides modest "retirement dollar support" for American workers. The Medicare program is age-related; once persons are 65, they are eligible for select medical coverage. Coverage is *incomplete* in two aspects, however: personal dollar contribution is mandatory and, moreover, long-term care health care services like skilled nursing facilities or home health services are covered only in limited circumstances. Means-tested Federal subsidies in the form of Supplemental Security Income and Medicaid are available to retired persons if their retirement financial resources are poverty-level or below or fall to such a level.

Financial subsidies for retirees cannot, as a rule, fully replace working income and fringe benefits. They only meet some living expenses and cover a variable portion of medical expenses. Despite the availability of pensions, personal savings (if any), and federal subsidies, retirement has a strong diminishing effect on income. Retirees of lower socio-economic status are generally more vulnerable to this effect.

# Chapter II

## RETIREMENT AND HEALTH
## FOR OLDER MEN

Much of the retirement literature in the past twenty years discuss retirement as a highly stressful experience for older men. High stress levels often relate to poor physical and mental health, and this relationship provides one reason for this current examination of retirement's effects. Chapter II begins with a discussion of why retirement negatively affects mental health. Retirement adjustment and retirement's unsatisfactory impact upon life satisfaction are examined in the beginning sections. The next major section concerns the physical health of older men, and why stress is related to poor physical health. The chapter concludes with a review of knowledge gaps in the research literature of the past 25 years concerning retirement and health.

## Impact of Retirement on Mental Health

### Retirement Adjustment

"Retirement adjustment" is a very loosely defined term that has many meanings that depend upon the theoretical base used in the specific research (MacBride, 1976). The definition of "good adjustment" is uncertain due to an inconsistency in the scaling of adjustment measures. One study has presented retirement adjustment as a concept synonymous with life satisfaction (Peppers, 1976). This current study conceptualizes retirement adjustment as a *process* whose outcome can be *measured* in terms of life satisfaction.

The retirement adjustment process is influenced by health, income, pre-retirement attitudes, and the "time factor." One version of the "time factor" is introduced by Goudy and Reger (1985) who report that retired men find retirement to have been worse in expectation then in reality. Thus, retirement attitudes change positively with time, and poor retirement adjustment seems less likely. In contrast, MacBride (1976) interprets "the time factor" as important when retirement is examined at different points in post-retirement life. She states that the level of observed retirement adjustment depends on how soon after retirement the retiree is observed.

Despite many reports of good retirement adjustment, some research convincingly reports that one-third of all retirees have difficulty adjusting to retirement (Atchley, 1982). After all, retirement forces men to end personal involvement in their work lives and to attend to their new retired lives. This change brings with it demands for adjustment.

Older men, who have worked most of their adult lives and have depended upon traditional marriages and relationships, find adjusting their lives to this new retired role to be stressful. Retired men, who (1) are no longer married, (2) do not have a confidant, or (3) are not involved in community activities, find it particularly difficult to adjust (Antonucci, 1983; Palmore, 1976; Guttman, 1978; Cameron and Persinger, 1983; Fillenbaum, 1971). Moreover, when men have no choice in determining when and how to retire, their ability to cope is hindered. This also raises the probability of an unsuccessful adjustment. A number of researchers find *poor* retirement adjustment to be associated with poor health, low income and lack of personal resources, the inappropriate timing of retirement, lack of meaningful activities, and low marital satisfaction (Jackson and Gibson, 1983; Parnes and Nestel, 1981; Palmore, 1985; Atchley, 1976).

To help alleviate retirement adjustment difficulties, these difficulties should be examined in light of *other* adjustment problems in the retiree's life (Maddox, 1970). Maddox feels retirees may not be reconciling pre-retirement beliefs and attitudes (developed as young adults) with post-retirement circumstances. He suggests a problem-solving technique that involves assessment of the retiree's personality, life history, income, health. Such problem-solving will facilitate retirement adjustment and, thus, will give service-providers information about the retiree's satisfaction with his life as a whole.

## Retirement Affects the Life Satisfaction of Older Men

"Life satisfaction" is the psychological state men experience when they assess the overall condition of their life-as-a-whole and then compare their aspirations with their achievements (Baur and

Okun, 1983). This conceptualization of life satisfaction is especially apropos for retired men in America because for them achievement is a cultural imperative: "men must be successful." "True success" is generally characterized by a profitable and consistent worklife. Because retirement generally means that work has ceased, unhappiness with retirement contributes to life dissatisfaction (Guttman, 1978).

Research findings suggest that adults' mental health when measured by life satisfaction may increase as they age (Rodgers and Converse, 1976). However, this may be an overly optimistic assessment when one considers retired men. Other research points out that this increase in life satisfaction is probably contingent on several crucial factors including frequency of stressful life events, income, education, current physical health and prior mental health (Kremer, 1985; Robinson et al., 1985; Atchley, 1976; Palmore, 1964; Parnes and Nestel, 1981; Bradford, 1979). These factors are very variable in older adult populations but are often negative influences for their life satisfaction.

Retirement stress and the stigma attached to being old in America affect retirees' life satisfaction negatively. Retirees' life satisfaction is the subject of Guttman's research (1978) and he analyzes what he sees as two general categories of retirees: "action-takers" and "rocking-chair retirees." He describes action-takers as retirees who have high life satisfaction and who seek to maintain control of their lives. Action-takers are likely to use satisfactory coping techniques when stressful situations arise. Alternatively, rocking-chair retirees are men who are relatively helpless in times of stress because the coping skills of action-takers are unknown to them.

The situation of rocking-chair retirees requires closer scrutiny than that of action-takers because rocking-chair retirees represent that minority of retirees who need clinical intervention to help them deal with retired life. Social isolation—the absence of social ties and relationships—is a common characteristic of rocking-chair retirees. Unfortunately, this lack of social relationships is a particularly important determinant of life dissatisfaction among rocking-chair retirees (Cutrona et al., 1986; Levitt et al., 1982). The favorable circumstances which predispose action-takers to good life satisfaction (such as sturdy social support systems and knowledge of problem-solving skills) are missing from the lives of the rocking-chair retirees.

# Impact of Retirement on Physical Health

## Physical Health

Minkler (1981a) reports that the physical health effects of retirement are uncertain. However, it is true that the aging process has a general *negative* effect on physical health and, thus, older adults display patterns of physical health problems. Wan et al. (1982) itemize these problems in a national study of 1182 older adults: 86 percent have chronic ailments such as arthritis, 38 percent need assistance with personal activities of daily living as a result of deteriorated health, 33 percent have trouble getting around because of disabilities, 29 percent are confined to their homes because of mobility problems, and 8 percent have trouble with self-maintenance because of malfunctions with important body processes. These findings are supported in similar research by Ford (1981) and Shanas and Maddox (1983).

Besides being more susceptible to diseases, older persons are also more physically vulnerable to stressful events such as retirement (and death of a spouse/significant other), as Parnes and Nestel (1981) report. Although the retirement literature is inconclusive, there *is* evidence that retirement can negatively affect physical health (Stokes and Maddox, 1967; Maddox and Douglas, 1973; Atchley, 1976; Haynes et al., 1977). With the certainty that the retirement rate will be *increasing* for the next 40 years, the likelihood of an increase in number of retired men with physical health problems is certain.

While there is a reasonable certainty for increased morbidity in the older population, Rabin (1984) reports statistics that indicate *declines in the mortality rate* of all adults aged 65 and older between 1950 to 1980. Moreover, it is interesting to note that, when the older adult population is divided into three groups that are 65 to 74 years old, 75 to 84 years old, and 85 years and older, the greatest overall decline in death rate is for those 85 and older. The second greatest decline in death rate is for those 65 to 74 years old, and this cohort is the most numerous among the aged.

Rabin says that this trend will assure a continued accumulation of those 85 years and older for the remainder of this century. He makes this prediction based on declining death rates for cardiovascular diseases, cancers, and respiratory diseases for the population aged 65 years and older. According to Rabin, the decrease is associated with increased access and use of medical services because of Medicare as well as improved medical technology.

However, Wylie (1984) has looked at differences in disease-specific death rates of elderly men versus elderly women in the United States. He reports faster declines in female death rates for cardiovascular diseases that have caused a wide gap between male and female death rates. Males have always had a higher death rate than females in all age groups, but the death rate for males has not been decreasing as rapidly as it has been for females in recent decades. Data for 1980 indicate a *greater rate of male mortality* for the three major causes of death (cardiovascular illness, cancers, and respiratory illnesses) in addition to accidents, homicide, and suicide.

## Theory Linking Stress to Poor Physical Health

The human body initially reacts to stressful life events by triggering damaging emotional states that stimulate autonomic nervous system activity. The body later undergoes harmful physiological changes, e.g. glandular disturbances and vascular constriction that can lead to heart disease, and ulcers. The theory behind this chain-of-events can be traced to the second half of the nineteenth century. Selye (1974) writes that French biologist Claude Bernard discussed the natural ability of the human body to resist disease by maintaining its own balanced *milieu interieur*.

Selye reports that this theory was further developed by German psychiatrist Adolf Meyer in 1910, who revealed that this internal equilibrium can be prone to *disequilibrium*. The results of his case studies show that people become ill after they experience stressful life events. What Meyer's work suggests is that the psychological impact of these events disrupts the body's defense system and increases susceptibility to diseases.

Since the 1950s, researchers such as Wolf (1981), Holmes and Rahe (1967), Selye (1974), Cassel (1976b), and Preston and Mansfield (1984) have reported that stress is a precursor of illness. Wolf says that life events and emotional states are related to specific diseases. Using Wolf's work as a base, Holmes and Rahe studied the stress/illness relationship extensively. They designed the "Social

Readjustment Rating Scale" as a classic instrument to predict stress-related illnesses. Preston and Mansfield (1984) have recently examined stress with sample of 200 elderly. One-quarter of their sample live "stress-free" lives and have good physical health. However, the remaining 75 percent of the sample have highly stressful lives, low levels of subjective health, and high levels of physical limitations.

## Gaps in the Research Literature
## on Retirement and Health

The literature generally reports that poor physical and mental health is often the case when men cannot cope with stress (Preston and Mansfield, 1984; Levitt et al., 1984; Cassel, 1976b; Hansson, 1986; Checkoway, 1988; Minkler, 1988; Israel, 1988). An examination of the retirement/stress/health literature reveals knowledge gaps, nonetheless. Empirical studies commonly focus on broader adult samples of both sexes when examining the relationships between stressful life events such as retirement and death of a spouse/significant other, and physical and mental health. Few studies look only at older men, and fewer studies look at men in the context of retirement and death of a spouse/significant other as stressful life events.

Moreover, research literature written in the past twenty-five years concerning the relationships between retirement and physical/mental health has been inconclusive. Cross-sectional "retirement and health" research studies are major contributors to this literature. Atchley (1976) and Haynes et al., (1977) have done cross-sectional analyses of retirement effects, and have concluded that retirees have poorer physical and mental health than non-retirees. Haynes et al., emphasize the role of the breakdown and loss of social contacts among retirees, and they conclude that suicide motivation and affective disorders are more prevalent in the retired population. All of the studies mentioned *do not* control pre-retirement characteristics.

However, research scientists recently have understood this failure to control pre-retirement characteristics as a methodological weakness and have questioned the accuracy of these findings. Longitudinal studies *can* control for pre-retirement characteristics such as physical health or income, and this study-type has become clearly preferred over cross-sectional studies. In a national longitudinal study, Parnes and Nestel (1981) eliminate those men who retired for poor physical health from their experimental sample, and find that retirement has little or no effect on physical health. They have also done analyses of other major national longitudinal studies—the Retirement History Study, the Panel Study of Income Dynamics, and the National Longitudinal Study. Parnes and Nestel conclude that retirement's effects are influenced by the prior job itself and retirement's timing. Retirement only indirectly affects mental health outcomes.

Mental health effects of retirement are difficult to isolate from physical health effects, as Minkler (1981b) discovered when she studied the latter. Because of their overlap, she feels retirement must be studied longitudinally with a psychosocial perspective to get a more reliable picture of its effects. A psychosocial framework would consider physical health, psychological health, and socio-economic factors as pre-conditions and outgrowths of this stressful life event. Such considerations have been used in developing the theoretical model for this current study that is discussed in the next chapter.

## Chapter III

## A SUGGESTED THEORETICAL MODEL

Men's retirement as a stressful life event that causes poor physical and mental health is the main focus of this research. Death of a spouse/ significant other is examined as an additional stressful life event that raises a retired man's already elevated stress level by robbing him of his closest provider of support. To these ends, a broad theoretical framework is used that explains the relationship between stress, as the causal agent, and poor physical and mental health as outcomes. Within this framework, the research argument uses three important factors as theoretical links in this relational sequence: the social environment, social support, and self-esteem.

### Variables to be Included in the Model

The theoretical model created for this study (see Figure 1) indicates that stressful life events directly affect physical and mental health. The measured variables used for this research are retirement, death of a spouse/ significant other, and physical and mental health. This theoretical model illustrates the testable hypothetical model in this study, and also shows untestable but relevant relationships.

Self-esteem and social support are crucial elements in the modeled processes, but they are not measured in these data. However, they are strongly implied, and their relationships to the measured variables are important. These relationships include: (1) the relationship between the personal loss men experience in these stressful life events and the subsequent reduction of their self-esteem levels; and (2) the relationship between these stressful life events and men's coping ability when they have a poor support system or none at all.

Premises of this study include: low self-esteem increases susceptibility to poor physical health; unsatisfactory social support reduces an older man's self-esteem and this can lead to poor physical health; and older men develop poor physical health when they are not satisfied with social support received and, thereby, feel extremely stressed.

*23*

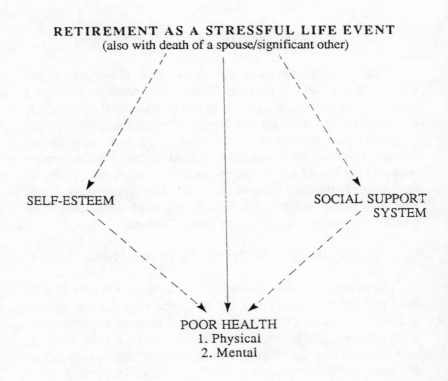

RETIREMENT AS A STRESSFUL LIFE EVENT
(also with death of a spouse/significant other)

SELF-ESTEEM                                          SOCIAL SUPPORT
                                                        SYSTEM

POOR HEALTH
1. Physical
2. Mental

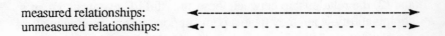

measured relationships:
unmeasured relationships:

**Figure 1. Theoretical Model.**

# Theoretical Relationships of
# Variables in the Model

This current research draws its theoretical foundations from related research that holds that social environmental factors can be *risk* factors in the lives of adults and endanger physical and mental health (Cassel 1976a; Heller et al., 1986). Such research is modeled around the concept of multifactorial causation in which the outcome is a function of several precipitating factors that are related (Heller et al. 1986). The theoretical conceptualization that influence this current model depicts stressful life events as social environmental changes that have negative effects on levels of self-esteem, social support, and physical and mental health.

Two important aspects of this theoretical framework are *not* measured in this study: negative changes in self-esteem and in social support systems. The fact that these changes are assumptions represents a methodological weakness of this longitudinal research, and a real limitation of secondary analysis. However, it is fortunate that literature supports these relationships. For example, Atchley (1976) states the retirement frequently causes negative changes in men's social systems. These negative changes can jeopardize men's ability to cope with the stress of retirement (Kessler, 1982; Coyne and DeLongis, 1986). Social support systems composed of spouse, family, and friends all have the potential of rupturing because of retirement-related stress.

Retirement-related stress also wears upon men's self-esteem (Elwell and Maltbie-Crannell, 1981; Sells, 1070; Bradford, 1979; Palmore et al., 1975; Eisdorfer, 1972; Nadelson, 1969; Quinn, 1981). Retirement often forces men to live the remainder of their lives in social-isolation if they are single. If they have families, these retired men are no longer the major provider. Self-esteem suffers.

Heller et al., (1986) say that social support embodies the basic social processes that enhance self-esteem and adjustment to stressful life events. In particular, they point out that *the* important aspect of social support to help accomplish health maintenance is its esteem-enhancing potential. For these reasons, this current research finds it important to look at social support in the stress and coping contexts of retirement and death of a spouse/significant other. This current research departs from traditional methodologies by focusing on the *one* component of the social support process that is usually not tested—*satisfaction* with social support. This new methodology is supported by Heller et al., who emphasize that to determine social support's effectiveness "the concept of social support needs to be disaggregated into component processes, and that the effects of social support on health outcomes can be best measured by gauging *satisfaction* with support." This current work uses that methodology.

## Mental and Physical Health Effects
## of the Social Environment

There is extensive literature concerning relationships between social environment and mental and physical health (Cutrona et al., 1986); Heller et al., 11986; House et al., 1982; Schaefer et al., 1981; Wallston et al., 1983; and Wolf, 1981). Until recently, researchers saw the social environment only as a source of stress. Now, however, some researchers report that a change in one's social environment possibly may benefit an individual.

Cassel (1976b) speaks about the possible role of social and cultural stress factors as determinants of disease. He says man is a social animal; social needs are as important as biological ones. For instance, when a man finds his work environment to be stressful and he has the opportunity and choice to plan his retirement, his new life as a retiree may prove to alleviate much of his work-related stress. Stress-related illnesses are now less likely to develop because such men can use the social environment as a resource to mediate the relationship between stress and physical and mental health.

While there is no clear-cut understanding of how the social situations in one's social environment can be health protective, some controlled empirical research has shown that persons with meaningful social systems in their social environment have significantly more favorable mental and physical outcomes than those with none (House et al., 1982; Antonucci and House, 1983; Minkler, 1981b; Lin et al., 1979; Wolf, 1981; Checkoway, 1988, Israel, 1988, Minkler, 1988).

However, Cassel (1976) points out that social situations may be characterized by any number of factors that may be potentially harmful. First, individuals may experience a new social situation like retirement, and the outcomes may be uncertain. Second, personal reactions to this uncertainty may be ones of "flight" or "fright." In either case, constructive coping with the situation has thus been avoided. Cassel considers both responses to be detrimental to well-being and physical health. Third, a positive outcome may be dependent upon the constant attention of the individual to the situation, and this process may be stressful for a retired man. He may lack material, physical or emotional resources to contain or reduce the stress. In general, Cassel cites that social disorganization like this is harmful for physical health, even when socio-economic status is controlled.

## Self-esteem, Social Support and Physical and Mental Health

### Theoretical Importance of Self-esteem

The study of whether supportive social systems in a man's social environment help him to cope with stressful life events such as retirement and death of a spouse/ significant other has not been exhaustive (Kessler, 1982). However, it is important to point out that researchers have determined that self-esteem is crucial when social relationships act as buffers for stressful life events in older men's lives (Lieberman, 1986; Thoits, 1986).

A man's self-esteem level vacillates as stressful events wear upon his mental health. Self-esteem in older men may thus depreciate considerably, especially when retirement or death of spouse/ significant other causes sudden negative changes in their social system. As older men continue to suffer reduced self-esteem levels and their social ties become fewer, these men can become socially isolated. Their entire lives are dramatically affected by these life events. It is no surprise that Palmore (1976) finds a positive relationship between low self-esteem and poor mental health.

The work by Antonucci and Jackson (1983) establishes a strong relationship between self-esteem and self-reported physical health. They report a significant correlation between low self-esteem and health problems, although the causal direction could not be determined. However, they suggest this question: Are people with low self-esteem more prone to illness?

Extrapolating from their findings to the context of the life events used in this research, one asks about the relationship between men's retirement as a stressful life event and their self-esteem. If low self-esteem is an outcome of retirement or at least associated with it, can it then be assumed that these men will experience poor physical health? Moreover, while low levels of self-esteem may predispose men to poor physical health, can low levels of self-esteem also negatively affect good health behaviors?

Such negative health behavior change has the potential to lead to illness behavior and, ultimately, poor physical health. Nevertheless, Antonucci and Jackson deduce that self-esteem, most likely, has a reciprocal relationship with physical and mental health problems. Thus, low self-esteem can either cause or result from poor physical health. In the context of this current research, low self-esteem is thought to be a product of stressful life events and negatively influences retired men's physical health.

## Theoretical Importance of Social Support

As discussed extensively in Chapter I, researchers report that when older male retirees have effective personal social support systems operating in their lives, their physical and mental health is generally good (Checkoway, 1988; Israel, 1988; Minkler, 1988). There are two main reasons for this relationship. First, these older men actively maintain their social ties despite the fact that they have retired and/or have lost a spouse or significant other through death. These social processes help them to change the meaning of the stressful events and help them to cope. Second, the social processes act to induce good self-esteem in them and to contribute to their satisfaction with their overall life.

Social support is transmitted to an individual by what Levitt et al., (1982) refer to as a convoy, that is, a group of persons who are connected to the individual via the giving (or receiving) of social support. Social support can assist older retirees to cope with life events in several ways depending upon the circumstances. Retirees could receive emotional support (like love or caring); they could receive more focussed help such as cognitive restructuring (correcting irrational thought patterns); or they could receive instrumental aid like money or food (Cutrona et al., 1986).

Satisfaction with the support received and with potential support is an important determinant of good physical and mental health outcomes for elderly persons, much more so than quantity or frequency of social support (Antonucci and House, 1983). Antonucci and House find that spouses are the most satisfactory source of social support for older individuals. Levitt et al., (1982) further specify this concept by revealing that men generally have no extended network and tend to rely heavily on the spouse relationship. Older men are particularly dependent on their spouses for much of their emotional support before and after retirement; satisfaction with spouse-support is crucial for the good mental health of older, retired men.

When men retire and are both *old* and *sick*, social support from spouses can have a very positive effect and improve physical health. Because these men's situation is "normative or expected in their life cycle," Antonucci and House (1983) claim that spouse social support acts as an ameliorative measure. However, if a spouse is not available, support from a significant other may not be as significantly positive because of the cultural mores that exist in America. Hence, as pointed out earlier, many retired men have no source of support other than their spouse. Other family members or close friends represent untouched personal resources that can help meet some of the needs of older men. Levitt et al., (1982) report that independent and self-sustaining men lack the necessary social support needed to allay fears of dependence on an American impersonal health care system.

The theoretical model and framework discussed in this chapter provide the rationale for this research. The next chapter utilizes this retirement research and the newly developed theoretical model as guidelines for the methodological design of this current research that seeks to contribute to social science knowledge.

Chapter IV

## METHODOLOGY

### The Hypotheses

The basic research question for study is: "What is the effect of retirement on the physical and mental health of this sample of older men?" Men's retirement is influenced by prior physical health and physical functioning, income while working, age and education. In turn, men's retirement later influences their *current* physical health and physical functioning, satisfaction with health, life satisfaction, and income education. All these factors will be examined in this exploratory study by taking two hypotheses into consideration.

The *first hypothesis* states that retirement is a stressful life event and is harmful for the physical and mental health of older men. The *second_hypothesis* states that when another stressful life event—death of a spouse/significant other—occurs to older men within the same four-year period as retirement, their physical and mental health becomes especially problematic, moreso than if such a death occurs when men are working.

The variables in this research are drawn from questions in a two-wave project called "Social Networks in Adult Life," (Kahn and Antonucci, 1980, Survey Research Center, University of Michigan) and a 1984 follow-up by the same investigators called "Cancer Symptoms in the Elderly." The questions used in this current study are ones that appear in the first wave of the original project and are repeated *almost entirely* in the second wave of the project. The slight discrepancy appears in the physical health measures. (Please refer to the later section of this chapter dealing with physical health measures to learn about the differences between the physical health measures of 1980 and those of 1984.) Personal characteristics are used as control variables: age, education (1980), and income (1980) and (1984), as well as prior physical health (1980). Physical health and income data are available for 1980 and 1984; changes in physical health and income will be important features of this study.

The hypotheses are designed so that this study uses control

*31*

measures (prior physical health, income, age and education) measured at time "1" (T1) and outcome variables measured at time "2" (T2). This design determines the longitudinal character of the analysis. It will be interesting to examine the analyses resulting from this ordering of variables.

Moreover, the recency with which the two life events have occurred to men in this study is critical to their effects. The more recently retirement and death of a spouse/significant other have occurred, the more stressful they are assumed to be (Holmes and Rahe 1967). In this study, these events will have occurred within a *four*-year period and should be recent enough to qualify as stressful. Thus, older men are being studied in the "double-stress" context of two life events.

## The Sample of Men

The sample of men (see Table 1) is derived from the aforementioned research project. The sample of *152 men* analyzed in this study are all the men in the 1984 study, and represent those who are retired as well as those who are not retired. The men who participated only in the 1980 phase of the study are not of interest because no data are available about them for 1984.

This sample has been drawn from a national sample of 1500 adults ranging in age from 50 to 88 that make up the original pool of subjects. In the first stage of the sampling design in 1980, the entire subject pool was given a 10-15 minute telephone interview about basic demographics, social support and well-being. Out of this sample, 718 adults 50 years and older participated in an in-depth interview regarding health and well-being.

Four hundred and four (404) of the 718 individuals interviewed in the second stage of the original data collection, 65 percent of the living members of that sample, were re-interviewed in 1984 for the second wave of the study using a computer-assisted telephone interviewing system. The 152 men used for this current research come from this pool of individuals. Some members of this sample of 152 men have retired and have also experienced the death of a spouse/ significant other. Women have been excluded from this study because not enough of them identified themselves as retired to permit systematic analysis.

The sample of 152 men is tested by statistical analysis to ascertain the effects of recent, potentially stressful life events (retirement and death of a spouse/significant other) on their current physical and mental health. Physical health will cover both relatively objective reports and more subjective appraisals. Mental health will be assessed by self-reports of satisfaction with life and satisfaction with physical health.

## Table 1. Retired Sample Description.
### Retired sample N = 48 men*

| Age range = 63 to 97 years | |
|---|---|
| Death of spouse = 3 men | Education range = 1 to 17+ gr |
| Death of significant other = 31 men | Mode of grade range = 10th |
| Income range 1980 = <br> <$5000 to $50,000+ | Income range 1984 = <br> <$5000 to $50,000+ |
| Income mode = $7500 | Income mode = $7500 |

\* Out of total sample, N = 152 men.

## Variable Measures

### Life Events

Retirement and death of a spouse/significant other are major predictors in this study. These events fall into the top half of the 43 potentially stressful life events listed in the self-report instrument Holmes and Rahe (1967) designed for a general adult population called the Social Readjustment Rating Scale. In fact, Holmes and Rahe consider death of a spouse to be the most stressful of all life events. Retirement is considered to be one of the ten most stressful life events.

The retirement and death of a spouse/significant other measures are taken from the following items in the 1984 questionnaires.

1. RETIREMENT [1984]: "Have you in the last four years retired from your job or major life occupation?"

2. WIDOWHOOD [1984]: "Have you in the last four years lost your husband/wife through death?"

3.  DEATH OF SIGNIFICANT OTHER [1984]: "Have you in the
    last four years experienced the death of some other close family
    member or friend?"

The three individual measures are dichotomous variables with
responses: yes, no, and have been dummy coded. In addition, the
widowhood and death of a significant other variables are additively
collapsed into a new single dichotomous variable called the "death of
a spouse/significant other" variable that indicates, yes: the respondent has lost a family member or friend by death; no: the respondent
has not.

In their research about life satisfaction issues, Campbell et al.,
(1976) have tested and have supported the accuracy of these life
event measures as reliable indicators of stress. Wolf (1981) offers
similar support. However, Preston and Mansfield (1984) suggest
that the scales measuring life event stress may not be able to accurately assess stress levels because they do not fully account for an
individual's perception of *poor physical health*. Preston and Mansfield claim that the stress of poor physical health is so strongly felt
by individuals affected that other life events which may occur will be
overpowered by their feelings of poor health. The experimental
sample in their study reports to them that physical health changes are
more stressful than *any other* life changes.

### Physical Health Measures

Physical health plays major roles in this study as a control
measure *and* as an outcome measure. Physical health in the elderly
population is best measured by assessing their *physical functioning*
as well as by considering the presence or absence of disease (World
Health Organization, 1959; Preston and Mansfield, 1984). A person's degree of fitness—the things he/she can do or thinks he/she
can do—is an appropriate indicator of how healthy he/she is, and
ultimately of what services he/she may require from the community.

Therefore, this analysis makes use of two types of physical
health measurements. First, the study uses physical health problem
indicators that are self-reports of physician treatments for illnesses
based on a self-selection of physical health problems from a given
list. Second, to measure functional ability, the study uses self-

assessment indicators of functional ability based on these scales—
Langley-Porter Physical Self-Maintenance Classifications (Lowenthal, 1964), and Instrumental Activities of Daily Living (Lawton and
Brody, 1969). However, the closed-ended physical health problems self-reports that are used in both time periods of this study are
problematic because of the ambiguity inherent in many answers. A
respondent could answer "yes" to having received treatment or
medication for stomach problems (indigestion, for example) while
someone else could respond "yes" to kidney problem (meaning
dialysis).

Consequently, the writer of this current study does not consider
these two responses comparable. The first could signify only some
discomfort; the second could mean serious   functional disability.
Moreover, a response to this question may not accurately reflect the
World Health Organization (1959) health definition used in this
study. Therefore, this study uses a physical health measure created
specifically for purposes of this analysis in which the health problems measure is additively indexed with measures of functional
ability. This construction process is described in the prior physical
health and current physical health sections that follow.

Maddox and Douglass (1973) find that this indexing of measurements produces reliable measures. In the case of older adults'
physical health, they assert that an elderly person's rating of his/her
physical health correlates positively with a physician's rating of the
person's physical health, and that self-rating of physical health is a
better predictor of future physician ratings than the reverse. The
technique of measuring individual physical health by indexing
relatively objective physical health-related reports with subjective
measures allows for a comprehensive assessment of physical health.

**Prior Physical Health.**    This research uses the prior
physical health measure from 1980 (T1) as a control measure. Past
empirical work shows that prior physical health is the most accurate
predictor of current physical health (Tausig, 1986). Consequently,
the effect of prior physical health on current physical health can be
made negligible if prior physical health is controlled. The effects of
the *main* predictors in this study (retirement and the death of a
spouse/significant other) can, therefore, surface as independent
effects that are free from other influences.

The original questions from the 1980 questionnaire that make up these individual physical health items are:

1. *Physical Health Problems*: "I'm going to read a list of health problems. After each one please tell me whether a doctor has given you treatment or medication for that problem in the past five years."

   (The respondent was asked to indicate whether he experienced any of the following: arthritis, stomach problems, ulcers, cancer, hypertension, diabetes, liver problem, kidney problem, stroke, blood circulation problem or hardening of the arteries, heart trouble, lung problem or trouble breathing, serious eye problem like glaucoma or cataracts, and hearing loss.)

2. *Other Serious Health Problems*: Do you have any serious health problems (that I haven't mentioned)? What are they?

   (A dichtomous variable—yes, no—was constructed by Kahn and Antonucci (1980) as the response to the first question. They categorized the answers to the second (open-ended) question as follows: non-serious physical symptoms, any other physical symptoms (serious), neurosis or psychosis, and drug addiction, lcoholism or cigarettes.)

3. *Personal and Functional Care Needs*: "Do you ever need anyone's help with your personal care needs, such as eating, bathing, dressing, or getting around the house/apartment?" and "How about taking care of other things such as shopping, driving, traveling, doing necessary business, taking care of the house—do you ever need anyone's help in taking care of these needs?"

   (Kahn and Antonucci created a three response index: yes, no, and temporary limitation. If the response was yes or temporary limitation, they asked an additional question, "How often do you need this type of help?" Again, they created a three response index: often, sometimes, and once in a while.)

The prior physical health measure used in this study is created by recoding the original responses to the three physical health questions. The first physical health problem question is close-ended. The second health problem question, however, is open-ended and must be recoded to categorize the responses into three levels of seriousness of other health problems. Then, both of these physical health questions are transformed so that the resulting single variable counts all the "yes" responses for health problems asked by the questions. Next, the personal and functional care needs questions are systematically transformed to isolate the "yes" responses in combination with the frequency of responses. Finally, these new forms of the physical health variables are additively transformed to create *one* measure that best indicates the quality of general physical health status of the respondents. This new variable represents the most accurate measure of the overall prior physical health status of these men.

**Current Physical Health.** Two physical health variables from the 1984 (T2) wave of this study have also been similarly re-coded and additively transformed to create a main outcome measure called "current physical health." As an outcome measure, "current physical health" is measured at T2 and is based on only two of the three identical questions regarding *physical health problems* and *functional care needs* that were used for prior physical health.

By additively transforming both physical health measures, these two variables are linked to best *assess* the current physical health of this sample according to Rodgers and Converse (1975). The open-ended disease question used at T1 was *not* repeated. (Please refer to questions #1 and #3 in the "prior physical health" description for the 1984 questionnaire items that constituted the physical health questions.)

## Mental Health Measures

Satisfaction with life and satisfaction with health are the components of mental health used in this research. Each concept is created by additively collapsing relevant questions from the original 1984 questionnaire. The two new variables are called "comprehensive life satisfaction" and "physical health satisfaction."

**Comprehensive Life Satisfaction.** Responses to the three following questions are used to form a scale called "comprehensive life satisfaction":

1.  How satisfied are you with your friendships, that is, the things you do with your friends, and how you get along with them?

2.  How satisfied are you with your family life—the time you spend and the things you do with members of your family?

3.  How satisfied are you with your life as a whole these days?

The three variables are additively indexed to form one new variable measuring comprehensive life satisfaction. For purposes of this study, the responses to the variables have been compressed from a seven point scale that reads: "completely dissatisfied, very dissatisfied, dissatisfied, neutral, satisfied, very satisfied, completely satisfied," to a five-point scale that reads: "completely dissatisfied, dissatisfied, neutral, satisfied, completely satisfied."

Compression of responses acts to increase the number of individuals in some of the "cells" and facilitates meaningful statistical analyses. This new single measure is designed to accurately measure comprehensive life satisfaction. Rodgers and Converse (1975) support the indexing of related life satisfaction variables and they state that there is encouraging evidence for the reliability and validity of these indexed measures. The "life as a whole" variable, when used singularly, has been shown to have poor reliability because the concept is too broad. "People are not used to referring to their situation in that way," according to Rodgers and Converse. They recommend that variables addressing certain features of life known as "domains of life" also be incorporated into a new larger measure to increase reliability.

Overall life satisfaction can be accurately measured by an additive combination of important domain-of-life variables. "Family" and "friends" are such domains. They are factors relevant to a large majority of the population and are responsive to necessary shifts in life situations due to death of a spouse, family member or friend. As well, the literature in Chapters 2 and 3 support their relationships to physical and mental health. The above relationships are especially meaningful in this current research because *changes* in retired men's life satisfaction due to death of a spouse/significant other are of interest.

This new comprehensive life satisfaction variable is thus conceptualized as the by-product of stressful life events effects and social support dissatisfaction. This conceptualization is an out-growth of literature and theory that has been discussed in the previous chapters of this study. Self-esteem levels, while not measured directly in this research, are strongly implied by these variables.

**Physical Health Satisfaction.** The "physical health satisfaction" variable is created by additively indexing the responses to two separate questions. Again, a more comprehensive single variable is wanted which, in this case, accurately reflects a fuller measurement of satisfaction with physical health. Each variable is originally composed of a seven-point interval scale identical to the comprehensive life satisfaction measures. The responses to each question have been reduced to the new five-point scale that has also been done with comprehensive life satisfaction. The two variables that make up this new physical health satisfaction variable are:

1) Please tell me how satisfied you are with your physical ability to do the things you *want* to do.

2) Overall, how satisfied are you with your health?

With this more encompassing measure, psychological reactions to these two questions, which overlap in content to some degree, are ascertained.

Rodgers and Converse (1975) would see this indexed physical health satisfaction measure as more reliable than any of each of its two separate components for two reasons. First, they suggest that use of specific domain measures such as "physical activity" allows respondents some ease in evaluating this factor. The "physical activity" question breeds more free-flowing responses because of its familiarity and specificity. Thus, Rodgers and Converse claim that the concept of "physical activity" is more frequently rehearsed and settled upon in the respondent's mind. Second, Rodgers and Converse say this sort of psychological measurement is reliable because *two* variables are being used to measure the *same* entity.

In this current study, relationships between retirement and physical and mental health are examined. Many prior retirement studies have been cross-sectional; this study is longitudinal and uses *two* measures of physical health which cover a nine year span. The diverse literature about retirement and health reflects the complexities inherent in an examination of those relationships. But when retirement *plus* death of a spouse/significant other are then considered, relational complexities increase even more. This study is designed to highlight changes taking place in objective (physical health) and subjective (mental health) conditions of older men's lives once they all have retired, as well as when some men have also experienced death of a spouse/significant other.

This current study is also different from other national longitudinal retirement studies in two respects. First, Parnes and Nestel (1981) are concerned in their study with the match between *pre-retirement* expectations and the *impact of retirement* upon quality of life, measured by sample responses concerned with happiness with life, standard of living, leisure, housing, and health. This study, however, is only concerned with *retirement's consequences* upon physical health and mental health (life satisfaction and physical health satisfaction). The only pre-retirement factors that are utilized in this study are prior physical health and demographics, and these factors are controlled. Second, while Parnes and Nestel find no pre- and post-retirement differences regarding quality of life, the current study hypothesizes that retirement generally has negative effects upon physical and mental health. Parnes and Nestel eliminate from their study those men who retired for poor physical health. They estimate that these men also had lower incomes and were less satisfied with life than those who retired for other reasons. However, it is difficult to determine from their study if there is any directional relationship between retirement, and life satisfaction and income. It will be interesting to see the results of this current study because the sequencing of variables here does permit speculations about retirement's effects on consequential life satisfaction.

# Chapter V

## ANALYSIS AND RATIONALE

The formal tests are done using Least Squares Regression Analyses. It will be especially important to see how controlling prior physical health and demographic variables affects the power of retirement and death of a spouse/significant other in predicting the measures of physical and mental health. Preliminary exploratory analysis is done using correlations.

The sample size in this study is relatively small (N = 152), and some of the variables have minimal distribution, such as loss of a spouse/significant other (see Table 1). This study is designed to ascertain *relationships* rather than *causality*, and accordingly, the levels of significance used in these analyses have been increased to include p < .10. This adjustment will allow the reader to have a greater awareness of a range of independent variables that may have effects on the dependent variables. Variables significant at p < .10 are designated as showing "trends of interest" rather than disqualifying them completely. Hence, this research will be as useful as possible to professionals in the field because of the breadth of its implications.

Using the *entire male sample* from 1984 (T2), N = 152, the analyses are set up for correlation and main effect regression predictions. The time-sequencing of the variables over the nine-year period of the study may suggest several directional associations when correlations are done. The associations involve physical health and income; both are measured at T1 and T2. Therefore, physical health and income changes for this male sample could be evident. Education is measured at T1 and is a fixed measure. Age is a continuous measure.

Prior physical health is controlled in the multiple regression analysis. It is possible that significant prior physical health effects in the correlations may be "whitewashed" when regressions are run with the same variables. This would point to the powerful influence of prior physical health.

Any significant *interactive* effects between retirement and death of a spouse/significant other, retirement and age, retirement and income (T1), and retirement and education upon the physical and mental health outcomes are carefully evaluated. These interactive effects are tested because, as suggested in the earlier chapters of this dissertation, these factors influence men's lives when they retire, perhaps differently than they would when they are working.

For instance, men's retirement generally coincides with their loss of function as a main family provider, and being a provider is tied to education and income. Because a higher level of education usually indicates men's higher earning power as workers, when education is modest and income level is low, retirement usually means a *reduction* of this low income. When one considers these negative dynamics to be operating within older men's lives, one could expect such men to experience hardships in American society.

The meaning of retirement to the low-income person in this study (see Table 1) is difficult to hypothesize with the limited information available. As previously discussed, it is clear, however, that retirement does mean a reduction of "liveable" income, whether or not the individual has savings. The literature hypothesizes that the retiree may receive a small pension or be forced to depend upon social security payments alone for expenses. Thus, he may no longer have the benefit of company-paid health insurance and is no longer as attentive to his health. The welfare state in America will aid retired persons who are destitute, but oftentimes while retirement causes loss of income, it may *not* act to reduce income enough to qualify one for government monetary assistance. Those men who find themselves destined to live the remainder of their lives with meager incomes, yet no welfare subsidy, are at risk for poor physical and mental health.

Although retirement usually means *less* income to persons of *all* income levels, it affects low-income people *differently* than high-income people. The high income person generally has a pension, substantial savings, and his financial future is assured despite the fact that he may have seen a decline in the actual amount of new revenue. This hypothesis is salient to the purposes of this study. This study will attempt to show that retirement is harmful to the well-being of most older men, but maybe moreso for low-income men.

However, the literature also hypothesizes that retirement may be beneficial to low-income male workers. Reduced retirement income may now represent for the first time a stable and regular, albeit, small income. This, in itself, may be a boon to their lives because income is not dependent on physically or mentally stressful work. Their physical and mental health may actually improve. Retirement can, therefore, negatively affect income, but even a reduction in the actual number of dollars received may be offset by other factors in the retired individual's life such as improvements in physical or mental health.

As men age and retire, they also become more likely to experience death of a spouse/significant other. The consequences of these events in American society can be very stressful to older men and can have serious effects upon their self-esteem and mental health. To wit, as this paper has illustrated earlier, when a retired man's potentially weakened sources of support are considered, and his spouse dies, there is likely going to be compounded difficulties, more than the additive effects of each life event. Thus, the interactions tested in this study are designed to reveal some contextual features concerning retirement (and death of a spouse/significant other) as seriously damaging events in older men's lives. This knowledge will ultimately be used to improve older men's physical and mental health as they age in America.

The multiple regression equations will take the following forms:

1. Retirement will be used with the control variables as the sole predictor for the physical health and mental health outcomes.

2. Retirement and death of a spouse/significant- other will be used with the retirement x death interactive term and control variables as predictors for the physical and mental health outcomes.

3. Retirement in interaction with income (T1) will be examined as a predictor of physical and mental health in two ways: first, with retirement plus controls in one analysis, and then with both retirement and death of a spouse/significant other plus controls.

4. Retirement in interaction with age will be examined as a predictor of physical and mental health in two ways: first, with retirement plus controls in one analysis, and then with both retirement and death of a spouse/significant other plus controls.

5. Retirement in interaction with education will be examined as a predictor of physical and mental health in two ways: first, with retirement plus controls in one analysis, and then with both retirement and death of a spouse/significant other plus controls.

## Chapter VI

## RESULTS AND DISCUSSION

### Does Retirement Significantly Predict
### Current Physical Health?

Examination of results from main regression analyses of this study reveals no significant predictive relationships involving men's retirement (Table 2) or men's retirement in interaction with death of a spouse/significant other (Table 3) to their current physical health. When retirement plus prior physical health, age, income at T1 and T2, and education are tested by multiple regression analyses as predictors of current physical health, neither retirement or retirement in interaction with death of a spouse/significant other, surfaces as a significant predictor of negative physical health as hypothesized. The only factor that is a significant positive predictor of current physical health is prior physical health.

When the retirement x income (T1) interaction (Table 4), the retirement x education interaction (Table 5), and the retirement x age interaction (Table 6) are analyzed separately, the same result appears. Neither retirement nor retirement in interaction with these social factors are significant predictors; prior physical health remains the only significant positive predictor for current physical health.

Furthermore, when death of a spouse/significant other is included in the predictive equations, none of the other interactive terms—retirement x income (T1) in Table 7, retirement x education in Table 8, or retirement x age in Table 9—has any significant negative effect regarding the physical health of these men. Thus, retirement does *not* significantly predict harmful physical health outcomes for men in the sample when these social factors interact with retirement and death of a spouse/significant other. This conclusion supports similar findings of other longitudinal studies (Palmore, et al., 1979; Parnes and Nestel, 1981).

All of these predictive analyses are done controlling (for) men's prior physical health, age, income at T1 and T2, and education. Nevertheless, despite the fact that retirement is *not* a significant pre-

## Table 2

Multiple Regression Analysis of Retirement Plus the Control Variables as Predictors for Current Physical Health.

Least Squares Regressions:                 testing the <u>male</u> sample, N = 152

Outcome Variable: Cur Phy Hlt (T2)

| Predictor Variable | b | part r | beta |
|---|---|---|---|
| Retirement (T2) | -.08 | -.02 | -.02 |
| <u>Controlling for:</u> | | | |
| Prior Physical Health(T1) | .55*** | .48 | .49 |
| Age(T1) | -.01 | -.06 | -.06 |
| Income(T1) | -.12 | -.09 | -.12 |
| Income(T2) | .14 | .11 | .15 |
| Education(T1) | .03 | .06 | .06 |
| Intercept | | 28.8 | |
| R | | .52 | |
| R$^2$ | | | .28 |
| F ratio | | 7.45*** | |

* p < .10; ** p < .05; *** p < .01

## Table 3

Multiple Regression Analysis of Retirement, Death of a Spouse/ Significant Other, the Retirement x Death Interaction, Plus the Control Variables as Predictors for Current Physical Health.

Least Squares Regressions: testing the <u>male</u> sample, N = 152

Outcome Variable: Cur Phy Hlt (T2)

| Predictor Variable | b | part r | beta |
|---|---|---|---|
| Retirement (T2) | -.12 | -.02 | -.03 |
| Death of a Spouse/Significant Other | .36 | .08 | .08 |
| Retirement x  Death interaction | .11 | .01 | .01 |
| Controlling for: | | | |
| Prior Physical Health (T1) | .55*** | .48 | .49 |
| Age (T1) | -.01 | -.05 | -.05 |
| Income (T1) | -.12 | -.08 | -.12 |
| Income (T2) | .14 | .11 | .15 |
| Education (T1) | .03 | .06 | .06 |
| Intercept | | 24.01 | |
| R | | .54 | |
| $R^2$ | | .29 | |
| F ratio | | 5.74*** | |

* $p < .10$; ** $p < .05$; *** $p < .01$

## Table 4

Multiple Regression Analysis of Retirement, the Retirement x Income (T1) Interaction Plus the Control Variables as Predictors for Current Physical Health.

Least Squares Regressions:          testing the <u>male</u> sample, N = 152

Outcome Variable: Cur Phy Hlt (T2)

| Predictor Variable | b | part r | beta |
|---|---|---|---|
| Retirement (T2) | -.40 | -.04 | -.09 |
| Retirement x Income (T1) interaction | .07 | .04 | .09 |
| <u>Controlling for:</u> | | | |
| Prior Physical Health (T1) | .55*** | .48 | .49 |
| Age (T1) | -.01 | -.06 | -.06 |
| Income (T1) | -.16 | -.10 | -.15 |
| Income (T2) | .14 | .11 | .15 |
| Education (T1) | .03 | .07 | .06 |
| Intercept | | 28.8 | |
| R | | .52 | |
| $R^2$ | | .28 | |
| F ratio | | 6.37*** | |

* $p < .10$; ** $p < .05$; *** $p < .01$

# Table 5

Multiple Regression Analysis of Retirement, the Retirement x Education Interaction Plus the Control Variables as Predictors for Current Physical Health.

Least Squares Regressions:     testing the <u>male</u> sample, $N = 152$
Outcome Variable: Cur Phy Hlt (T2)

| Predictor Variable | b | part r | beta |
|---|---|---|---|
| Retirement (T2) | -.82 | -.05 | -.19 |
| Retirement x Education interaction | .06 | .05 | .18 |
| <u>Controlling for:</u> | | | |
| Prior Physical Health (T1) | .54*** | .47 | .49 |
| Age (T1) | -.01 | -.07 | -.06 |
| Income (T1) | -.13 | -.09 | -.13 |
| Income (T2) | .14 | .11 | .15 |
| Education (T1) | .02 | .04 | .04 |
| Intercept | | 30.88 | |
| R | | .52 | |
| $R^2$ | | .28 | |
| F ratio | | 6.39*** | |

* $p < .10$; ** $p < .05$; *** $p < .01$

## Table 6

Multiple Regression Analysis of Retirement, the Retirement x Age Interaction Plus the Control Variables as Predictors for Current Physical Health.

Least Squares Regressions:          testing the <u>male</u> sample, N = 152
                                    Outcome Variable: Cur Phy Hlt (T2)

| Predictor Variable | b | part r | beta |
|---|---|---|---|
| Retirement (T2) | 112.46 | .12 | 26.9 |
| Retirement x Age interaction | .05 | .12 | 26.9 |
| <u>Controlling for:</u> | | | |
| Prior Physical Health (T1) | .54*** | .48 | .49 |
| Age (T1) | -.29 | -.12 | -.12 |
| Income (T1) | -.09 | -.06 | -.09 |
| Income (T2) | .11 | .08 | .12 |
| Education (T1) | .03 | .06 | .06 |
| Intercept | | 58.2 | |
| R | | .53 | |
| R$^2$ | | .28 | |
| F ratio | | 6.70*** | |

* p < .10; ** p < .05; *** p < .01

## Table 7

Multiple Regression Analysis of Retirement, Death of a Spouse/ Significant Other, the Retirement x Income (T1) interaction Plus the Control Variables as Predictors for Current Physical Health.

Least Squares Regressions:     testing the <u>male</u> sample, N = 152

Outcome Variable: Cur Phy Hlt (T2)

| Predictor Variable | b | part r | beta |
|---|---|---|---|
| Retirement (T2) | -.51 | -.06 | -.12 |
| Death of a Spouse/Significant Other | .43 | .11 | .10 |
| Retirement x Income (T1) interaction | .10 | .05 | .12 |
| <u>Controlling for:</u> | | | |
| Prior Physical Health (T1) | .54*** | .48 | .49 |
| Age (T1) | -.01 | -.05 | -.04 |
| Income (T1) | -.16 | -.10 | -.16 |
| Income (T2) | .15 | .11 | .16 |
| Education (T1) | .03 | .06 | .06 |
| Intercept | | 22.84 | |
| R | | .53 | |
| $R^2$ | | .29 | |
| F ratio | | 5.80*** | |

* p < .10; ** p < .05; *** p < .01

## Table 8

Multiple Regression Analysis of Retirement, Death of a Spouse/ Significant Other, the Retirement x Education Interaction Plus the Control Variables as Predictors for Current Physical Health.

Least Squares Regressions:          testing the <u>male</u> sample, N = 152

Outcome Variable: Cur Phy Hlt (T2)

| Predictor Variable | b | part r | beta |
|---|---|---|---|
| Retirement (T2) | -1.10 | -.07 | -.26 |
| Death of a Spouse/Significant Other | .45 | .12 | .10 |
| Retirement x Education interaction | .08 | .06 | .25 |
| <u>Controlling for:</u> | | | |
| Prior Physical Health (T1) | .54*** | .47 | .49 |
| Age (T1) | -.01 | -.05 | -.05 |
| Income (T1) | -.13 | -.10 | -.13 |
| Income (T2) | .15 | .12 | .16 |
| Education (T1) | .02 | .03 | .03 |
| Intercept | | 25.50 | |
| R | | .53 | |
| $R^2$ | | .29 | |
| F ratio | | 5.83*** | |

* p < .10; ** p < .05; *** p < .01

## Table 9

Multiple Regression Analysis of Retirement, Death of a Spouse/ Significant Other, the Retirement x Age Interaction Plus the Control Variables as Predictors for Current Physical Health.

Least Squares Regressions:  testing the <u>male</u> sample, $N = 152$

Outcome Variable: Cur Phy Hlt (T2)

| Predictor Variable | b | part r | beta |
|---|---|---|---|
| Retirement(T2) | 100.98 | .11 | 24.11 |
| Death of a Spouse/Significant Other | .35 | .09 | .08 |
| Retirement x Age interaction | .05 | .11 | 24.2 |
| <u>Controlling for:</u> | | | |
| Prior Physical Health(T1) | .54*** | .48 | .49 |
| Age(T1) | -.02 | -.10 | -.10 |
| Income(T1) | -.09 | -.06 | -.09 |
| Income(T2) | .12 | .09 | .12 |
| Education(T1) | .03 | .06 | .06 |
| Intercept | | 50.4 | |
| R | | .54 | |
| $R^2$ | | .29 | |
| F ratio | | 6.00*** | |

* $p < .10$; ** $p < .05$; *** $p < .01$

dictor of negative physical health according to the regressions, it is important to realize that there *are* significant correlations in Table 10 between men's "prior" physical health at T1, retirement, and "current" physical health at T2. Tausig (1984) makes the same discovery when he finds prior physical health (T1) to be the best positive predictor of their current physical health at T2. In Table 10, retirement is positively correlated with good physical health before and *after* retirement. This is an important finding because it helps support this study's perspective concerning the meaning of retirement for older men.

What broad conclusions can be drawn from the results of the preliminary correlations and the main regressions? To illustrate some inferences, a reference is first made to the beginning of the methodology section where it is stated that the *ordering* of the variables in this two-wave study would be important. In that regard, it is noteworthy that retirement falls on the timeline *after* T1, but *before* current physical health at T2.

In this context, the main regression analysis has *not* found retirement to *negatively* influence current physical health at T2. As well, prior physical health has consistently been found to positively predict current physical health. In addition, the physical health of older men who have retired is good *prior* to retirement. The correlations also suggest retirement has not harmed these men's physical health. There seems to be a significant pattern from T1 when men are working, to the actual retirement event sometime later, and eventually to T2 when they have been living as retirees for a period of time. The consistency of that pattern is that the assessment of this sample's physical health remains constant.

What is then surmised as a result of these findings is that the retirement experience in these men's lives does *not appear* to be harmful to their physical health. Results *do not* indicate the negative consequences of retirement, and the significant results in Table 10 suggest the *opposite* trend. The hypothesis that retirement (with/ without death of a spouse/significant other) is harmful for older men's physical health is not reinforced. Rather, an implication of the results is that retirement *may* be beneficial for men's physical health. While, further research is necessary to determine and examine specific reasons for such beneficial effects, these findings reinforce conclusions of other national longitudinal retirement studies

Table 10. Correlation Matrix (N = 152).

| | Com Life Sat | Pr Phy Hlth | Retired | Death | Age | Inc 1 | Educ | Inc 2 | Phy Hlth Sat | Cur Phy Hlth |
|---|---|---|---|---|---|---|---|---|---|---|
| Com Life Sat | 1.0000 | | | | | | | | | |
| Pr Phy Hlth | .0682 | 1.0000 | | | | | | | | |
| Retired | .0693 | -.2129** | 1.0000 | | | | | | | |
| Death | .0900 | .0294 | .0137 | 1.0000 | | | | | | |
| Age | .1009 | -.1738* | .0250 | -.1119 | 1.0000 | | | | | |
| Inc 1 | .1229 | .1498* | .0710 | -.0181 | -.2745*** | 1.0000 | | | | |
| Educ | -.0501 | .0256 | .0338 | .0011 | -.0044 | .4440*** | 1.0000 | | | |
| Inc 2 | .0404 | .0497 | -.1273* | -.0242 | -.2824*** | .7351*** | .4370*** | 1.0000 | | |
| Phy Hlth Sat | .4027*** | .3140*** | -.1690* | .0038 | -.0052 | .1931** | .0275 | .1345* | 1.0000 | |
| Cur Phy Hlth | -.0559 | .5051*** | -.1538* | .1136 | -.1570* | .1066 | .0911 | .1337* | .3644*** | 1.0000 |

* p < .10; ** p < .05; *** p < .01

(Parnes and Nestel, 1981; Minkler, 1981b). The unique feature of this current research is that retirement and death of a spouse/ significant other were looked at jointly. However, they both showed no harmful effect upon physical health. This finding is an important contribution to the gerontological social science literature.

## Does Retirement Significantly Predict Comprehensive Life Satisfaction?

From Tables 11 and 12, we can see that neither retirement or retirement in interaction with death of a spouse/significant other influences comprehensive life satisfaction negatively. When retirement plus prior physical health, age, income at T1 and T2, and education are tested as predictors to comprehensive life satisfaction, retirement does *not* surface as a significant negative predictor. In fact, there are no significant negative predictors at all.

The analysis then includes each interaction term independently and the same result appears (Tables 13, 14 and 15). Retirement does *not* surface as a significant predictor of negative life satisfaction nor does any other variable. These results are consistent with Palmore's findings because he tests retirement and also finds it not to negatively affect mental health (Palmore, et al. 1979). Thus, retirement does not appear to be a harmful experience for the life satisfaction of older men. In all of the analyses, the inclusion of death of a spouse/ significant other in the predictive equation does not change the results (Tables 16, 17 and 18). The harmful "double-crisis" hypothesis leading to negative life satisfaction is *not* supported and that itself is an important finding. This finding acts to fill gaps in the literature that have found stress, and poor physical and mental health to be related to each other (Preston and Mansfield, 1984; Levitt, et al., 1984; Cassell, 1976b; Minkler, 1988). Moreover, it *contradicts* the premise of much of this literature and adds new knowledge to the field.

## Does Retirement Significantly Predict Satisfaction with Physical Health?

Men's retirement, as an independent measure, has no significant negative effect on their feelings of satisfaction with physical health (Table 19). When retirement plus prior physical health, age, income

## Table 11

Multiple Regression Analysis of Retirement, Plus the Control Variables as Predictors for Comprehensive Life Satisfaction.

Least Squares Regressions: testing the <u>male</u> sample, N = 152

Outcome Variable: Com Life Sat (T2)

| Predictor Variable | b | part r | beta |
|---|---|---|---|
| Retirement(T2) | .10 | .06 | .07 |
| Controlling for: | | | |
| Prior Physical Health (T1) | .03 | .08 | .08 |
| Age(T1) | .01* | .16 | .18 |
| Income(T1) | .07 | .14 | .22 |
| Income(T2) | -.9(-3) | -.001 | -.002 |
| Education(T1) | -.03 | -.13 | -.15 |
| Intercept | 32.05** | | |
| R | .25 | | |
| R² | .06 | | |
| F ratio | 1.29 | | |

* p < .10; ** p < .05; *** p < .01

## Table 12

Multiple Regression Analysis of Retirement, Death of a Spouse/ Significant Other, the Retirement x Death of a Spouse/Significant Other Interaction Plus the Control Variables as Predictors for Comprehensive Life Satisfaction.

Least Squares Regressions:        testing the <u>male</u> sample, N = 152

Outcome Variable: Com Life Sat (T2)

| Predictor Variable | b | part r | beta |
|---|---|---|---|
| Retirement (T2) | .07 | .03 | .04 |
| Death of a Spouse/Significant Other (T2) | | .13 | .07 |
| .08 | | | |
| Retirement x Death interaction | .10 | .03 | .04 |
| Controlling for: | | | |
| Prior Physical Health (T1) | .03 | .08 | -.08 |
| Age (T1) | .01* | .17 | .18 |
| Income (T1) | .08 | .14 | .22 |
| Income (T2) | .9(-3) | .001 | .002 |
| Education (T1) | -.03 | -.13 | -.15 |
| Intercept | | 33.6** | |
| R | | .27 | |
| $R^2$ | | .07 | |
| F ratio | | 1.17 | |

* p < .10; ** p < .05; *** p < .01

## Table 13

Multiple Regression Analysis of Retirement, the Retirement x Income (T1) Interaction Plus the Control Variables as Predictors for Comprehensive Life Satisfaction.

Least Squares Regressions: testing the <u>male</u> sample, N = 152

Outcome Variable: Com Life Sat (T2)

| Predictor Variable | b | part r | beta |
|---|---|---|---|
| Retirement(T2) | .29 | .08 | .19 |
| Retirement x Income(T1) interaction | -.04 | -.06 | -.15 |
| <u>Controlling for:</u> | | | |
| Prior Physical Health (T1) | .03 | .08 | .08 |
| Age(T1) | .01* | .16 | .17 |
| Income(T1) | .09* | .15 | .27 |
| Income(T2) | -.004 | -.008 | -.01 |
| Education(T1) | -.03 | -.13 | -.15 |
| Intercept | 32.0** | | |
| R | | .25 | |
| R$^2$ | | .06 | |
| F ratio | | 1.17 | |

* p < .10; ** p < .05; *** p < .01

## Table 14

Multiple Regression Analysis of Retirement, the Retirement x Education Interaction Plus the Control Variables as Predictors for Comprehensive Life Satisfaction.

Least Squares Regressions:            testing the male sample, N = 152

Outcome Variable: Com Life Sat (T2)

| Predictor Variable | b | part r | beta |
|---|---|---|---|
| Retirement(T2) | .51 | .08 | .34 |
| Retirement x Education interaction | -.03 | -.07 | -.29 |
| Controlling for: | | | |
| Prior Physical Health(T1) | .03 | .08 | .09 |
| Age(T1) | .01* | .17 | .18 |
| Income(T1) | .08* | .15 | .24 |
| Income(T2) | -.004 | -.008 | -.01 |
| Education(T1) | -.02 | -.09 | -.11 |
| Intercept | | 33.2** | |
| R | | .26 | |
| $R^2$ | | .06 | |
| F ratio | | 1.19 | |

* $p < .10$; ** $p < .05$; *** $p < .01$

## Table 15

Multiple Regression Analysis of Retirement, the Retirement x Age Interaction Plus the Control Variables as Predictors for Comprehensive Life Satisfaction.

Least Squares Regressions: testing the <u>male</u> sample, N = 152

Outcome Variable: Com Life Sat (T2)

| Predictor Variable | b | part r | beta |
|---|---|---|---|
| Retirement (T2) | 14.3 | .03 | 9.6 |
| Retirement x Age interaction | .007 | .03 | 9.5 |
| <u>Controlling for:</u> | | | |
| Prior Physical Health (T1) | .03 | .08 | .08 |
| Age (T1) | .01 | .12 | .15 |
| Income (T1) | .08 | .14 | .23 |
| Income (T2) | -.004 | -.008 | -.01 |
| Education (T1) | -.03 | -.13 | -.15 |
| Intercept | | 28.3 | |
| R | | .25 | |
| $R^2$ | | .06 | |
| F ratio | | 1.13 | |

\* p < .10; \*\* p < .05; \*\*\* p < .01

## Table 16

Multiple Regression Analysis of Retirement, Death of a Spouse/ Significant Other, the Retirement x Income (T1) Interaction Plus the Control Variables as Predictors for Comprehensive Life Satisfaction.

Least Squares Regressions:           testing the <u>male</u> sample, N = 152

Outcome Variable: Com Life Sat (T2)

| Predictor Variable | b | part r | beta |
|---|---|---|---|
| Retirement | .25 | .07 | .17 |
| Death of a Spouse/Significant Other (T2) .10 | | .16 | .10 |
| Retirement x Income(T1) interaction | -.03 | -.05 | -.12 |
| <u>Controlling for:</u> | | | |
| Prior Physical Health (T1) | .03 | .08 | .08 |
| Age (T1) | .01* | .17 | .18 |
| Income (T1) | .08* | .14 | .22 |
| Income (T2) | -.001 | -.003 | -.005 |
| Education (T1) | -.03 | -.13 | -.15 |
| Intercept | | 34.2** | |
| R | | .27 | |
| $R^2$ | | .07 | |
| F ratio | | 1.19 | |

* p < .10; ** p < .05; *** p < .01

## Table 17

Multiple Regression Analysis of Retirement, Death of a Spouse/ Significant Other, the Retirement x Education Interaction Plus the Control Variables as Predictors for Comprehensive Life Satisfaction.

Least Squares Regressions:　　　　testing the <u>male</u> sample, $N = 152$

Outcome Variable: Com Life Sat (T2)

| Predictor Variable | b | part r | beta |
|---|---|---|---|
| Retirement(T2) | .42 | .06 | .28 |
| Retirement x Education interaction | -.02 | -.05 | -.22 |
| Death of a Spouse/Significant Other (T2) | | .16 | .10 |
| .10 | | | |
| <u>Controlling for:</u> | | | |
| Prior Physical Health (T1) | .03 | .08 | .08 |
| Age (T1) | .01* | .18 | .19 |
| Income (T1) | .08* | .15 | .24 |
| Income (T2) | -.002 | -.004 | -.006 |
| Education (T1) | -.02 | -.10 | -.12 |
| Intercept | | 35.1** | |
| R | | .27 | |
| $R^2$ | | .07 | |
| F ratio | | 1.20 | |

* $p < .10$; ** $p < .05$; *** $p < .01$

## Table 18.

Multiple Regression Analysis of Retirement, Death of a Spouse/Significant Other, the Retirement x Age Interaction Plus the Control Variables as Predictors for Comprehensive Life Satisfaction.

Least Squares Regressions:            testing the <u>male</u> sample, N = 152

                                      Outcome Variable: Com Life Sat (T2)

| Predictor Variable | b | part r | beta |
|---|---|---|---|
| Retirement(T2) | 8.8 | .02 | 5.9 |
| Death of a Spouse/Significant Other (T2) | | .16 | .117 |
| .10 | | | |
| Retirement x Age interaction | .004 | .02 | 5.8 |
| Controlling for: | | | |
| Prior Physical Health (T1) | .03 | .07 | .08 |
| Age (T1) | .01 | .14 | .17 |
| Income (T1) | .08 | .14 | .23 |
| Income (T2) | -.001 | -.002 | -.004 |
| Education (T1) | -.03 | -.14 | -.15 |
| Intercept | | 32.0 | |
| R | | .27 | |
| $R^2$ | | .07 | |
| F ratio | | 1.16 | |

\* $p < .10$; \*\* $p < .05$; \*\*\* $p < .01$

## Table 19

Multiple Regression Analysis of Retirement Plus the Control Variables as Predictors for Physical Health Satisfaction.

Least Squares Regressions:  testing the <u>male</u> sample, N = 152

Outcome Variable: Phy Hlth Satis (T2)

| Predictor Variable | b | part r | beta |
|---|---|---|---|
| Retirement (T2) | -.24 | -.12 | -.12 |
| <u>Controlling for:</u> | | | |
| Prior Physical Health (T2) | .14*** | .26 | .26 |
| Age (T1) | .01 | .10 | .10 |
| Income (T1) | .10 | .14 | .14 |
| Income (T2) | .003 | .005 | .007 |
| Education (T1) | -.02 | -.07 | -.07 |
| Intercept | | 26.8 | |
| R | | .38 | |
| $R^2$ | | .14 | |
| F ratio | | 3.35*** | |

* $p < .10$; ** $p < .05$; *** $p < .01$

at T1 and T2, and education are tested as predictors of physical health satisfaction, retirement still does *not* surface as a significant predictor. The only factor that is a significant positive predictor of physical health satisfaction is actual *prior* physical health. When the retirement x death interaction is added, and the predictors are tested for effects, they also show *no* significant negative effect on physical health satisfaction (Table 20).

## A Significant Interactive Effect

A major finding is that the retirement x income (T1) interaction term is significant at the $p < .01$ level as a predictor for increasing physical health satisfaction (Table 21). A graph of this interaction (Figure 2) indicates that retirement can be beneficial for the physical health satisfaction of low-income men. It should be noted that income was measured at T1 when *these men were working*. Although this finding is counterintuitive, speculative explanations are not dealt with here.

This interaction suggests some interpretations of retirement's influence upon the physical health attitudes of low-income men. For *low-income retirees*, this study suggests retirement is extremely helpful for improving attitudes about their physical health and for probably boosting their mental well-being. For these men, retirement could mean a cessation of labor, more leisure time, or a secure income after retirement that is not dependent on the physical pressure of work. Now that they have more "time on their hands," they can attend to psychologically uplifting endeavors and perhaps be more attentive to their physical health. Retirement may very well represent a long-awaited reward to these men. Furthermore, low-income retirees may now have the benefits of Medicare or Medicaid for regular health care. Such attention to physical health can stabilize overall health and may lead to good health satisfaction.

Work attitudes and retirement attitudes can be important factors to consider in order to explain this interaction's significant result for low-income men. It is important to note that there is evidently a great contrast between work attitudes and retirement attitudes in low-income men. Work attitudes are generally negative. Low-income workers seems to be dissatisfied with many aspects of their jobs, e.g. salary, physical labor, long hours, monotony, etc. Their job

## Table 20

Multiple Regression Analysis of Retirement, Death of a Spouse/ Significant Other, the Retirement x Death Interaction Plus the Control Variables as Predictors for Physical Health Satisfaction.

Least Squares Regressions:     testing the <u>male</u> sample, N = 152

Outcome Variable: Phy Hlth Satis (T2)

| Predictor Variable | b | part r | beta |
|---|---|---|---|
| Retirement (T2) | -.14 | -.06 | -.07 |
| Death of a Spouse/Significant Other (T2) | | .13 | .05 |
| .06 | | | |
| Retirement x Death interaction | -.31 | -.07 | -.10 |
| <u>Controlling for:</u> | | | |
| Prior Physical Health (T2) | .14*** | .26 | .27 |
| Age (T1) | .01 | .11 | .11 |
| Income (T1) | .10 | .14 | .21 |
| Income (T2) | .003 | .005 | .008 |
| Education (T1) | -.02 | -.07 | -.08 |
| Intercept | | 29.3 | |
| R | | .39 | |
| $R^2$ | | .15 | |
| F ratio | | 2.5*** | |

* p < .10; ** p < .05; *** p < .01

## Table 21

Multiple Regression Analysis of Retirement, the Retirement x Income (T1) Interaction Plus the Control Variables as Predictors for Physical Health Satisfaction.

Least Squares Regressions:          testing the <u>male</u> sample, N = 152

Outcome Variable: Phy Hlth Satis (T2)

| Predictor Variable | b | part r | beta |
|---|---|---|---|
| Retirement(T2) | -.84** | -.19 | -.43 |
| Retirement x Income(T1) interaction | .14* | .16 | .37 |
| <u>Controlling for:</u> | | | |
| Prior Physical Health(T2) | .13*** | .26 | .26 |
| Age(T1) | .01 | .10 | .10 |
| Income(T1) | .03 | .04 | .07 |
| Income(T2) | .01 | .02 | .03 |
| Education(T1) | -.01 | -.06 | -.07 |
| Intercept | 26.9 | | |
| R | .41 | | |
| $R^2$ | .16 | | |
| F ratio | 3.3*** | | |

* p < .10; ** p < .05; *** p < .01

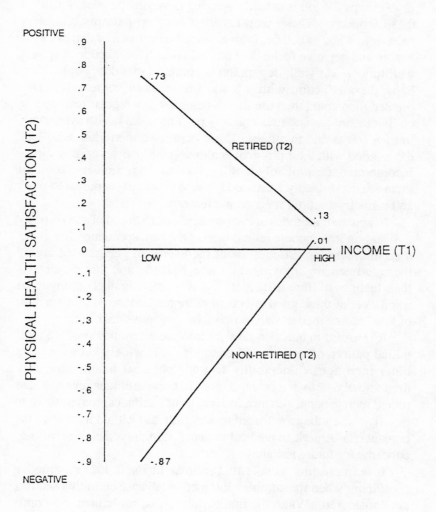

Figure 2. Retirement x Income (T1) Interaction with Physical
Health Satisfaction (N = 152).

negativity affects their sense of adequacy and, can have spinoffs in lowered physical health satisfaction.

Perhaps the job is actually wearing down the physical health of these workers. These workers then develop patterns of illness behavior. This, of course, is an expected outgrowth of deteriorating health, and negative feelings of physical health satisfaction may very well follow. As well, depression is common in older people. Perhaps, dissatisfaction with job and life leads to depression. Depressed men could then use illness behavior as a regular response or coping technique and thus magnify poor physical health symptoms to themselves and to others. These depressed men ultimately feel dissatisfied with their physical health as well. However, these low-income men are probably looking forward to retirement; some of them are undoubtedly frustrated because they must continue to work and cannot yet retire for economic reasons.

In contrast, attitudes about physical health are likely to be positive among low-income retired men. One can speculate that these men hold similar attitudes about their lives in general. Many of these retirees are enjoying their new lifestyle and this may boost their feelings of life satisfaction. As well, there is likely going to be a spillover of these good effects of retirement on the life satisfaction of low-income men to satisfaction with their physical health.

It is useful to question how far into the future this positive attitudinal pattern of retirees will continue. It is widely known that as older men age, vulnerability to poor physical health increases dramatically. At what point, if any, do these attitudes reverse? Do retired men generally change life and health attitudes from positive to negative when they are forced to seek help as sick old men from the bureaucratic American medical system? Certainly, these are serious concerns for future research.

It is interesting to note that retirement itself does emerge *as significant* when the complex interactions discussed in this section are considered. When the interaction terms, retirement x income (T1) [significant at the p < .05 level, Table 21] and retirement x education [significant at the p < .01 level, Table 22], are added separately, *retirement* is positively related to physical health satisfaction. These results seem limited to low-income men as the interaction indicates. The interaction is important despite being *contrary* to the first hypothesis that states that retirement is harmful

## Table 22

Multiple Regression Analysis of Retirement, the Retirement x Education Interaction Plus the Control Variables as Predictors for Physical Health Satisfaction.

Least Squares Regressions: testing the <u>male</u> sample, N = 152

Outcome Variable: Phy Hlth Satis (T2)

| Predictor Variable | b | part r | beta |
|---|---|---|---|
| Retirement (T2) | -1.2* | -.16 | -.65 |
| Retirement x Education interaction | .08 | .14 | .55 |
| <u>Controlling for:</u> | | | |
| Prior Physical Health (T2) | .13*** | .25 | .25 |
| Age (T1) | .01 | .09 | .09 |
| Income (T1) | .08 | .11 | .17 |
| Income (T2) | .01 | .01 | .02 |
| Education (T1) | -.03 | -.12 | -.13 |
| Intercept | | 23.9 | |
| R | | .40 | |
| $R^2$ | | .16 | |
| F ratio | | 3.2*** | |

* p < .10; ** p < .05; *** p < .01

for a mental health indicator like physical health satisfaction. This finding supports opposing research that claims retirement is a *beneficial* experience for the mental health of certain male retirees.

However, this effect is overpowered by the retirement x income (T1) interaction that is significant *only* with low-income men. The interaction result is important despite being *contrary* to the first hypothesis which states that retirement is harmful for a mental health indicator like physical health satisfaction because this finding supports research that claims retirement is a *beneficial* experience for the mental health of male retirees.

To the knowledge of this researcher, the relationships of retirement (and death of a spouse/significant other) to satisfaction with physical health have never been examined. Moreover, this study conceptualizes satisfaction with physical health as a component of mental health. In these novel and innovative contexts, research findings are bound to contribute new knowledge to the literature. To wit, this study has statistically linked the retirement experience to good physical health satisfaction for low-income men. Life satisfaction is a theoretical intermediary factor in this relationship. Retirement has been shown to be a *beneficial* experience especially for low-income men and this finding supports recent literature (Parnes and Nestel, 1981; Minkler, 1981b).

## Chapter VII

# IMPLICATIONS OF THE
# STUDY'S RESULTS

The results of this research show physical health, economic, and mental health factors are related in the pre- and post-retirement lives of older men. Moreover, the results imply that retirement is generally a beneficial experience for older men, the view of much of the contemporary literature (Parnes and Nestel, 1981; Minkler, 1981b). Prior physical health, age, income at T1 and T2, and education were controlled in *all* tests in this study.

Retirement was first studied here with controls as a single stressful life event that had hypothesized negative effects upon retired men's physical health because the experience of retiring wore upon their self-esteem and disrupted their social situations. This relationship was not substantiated by the data analysis. Retirement and the controls were then examined in interaction with age, education, income while working, and death of a spouse/significant other. Retirement was again found not to be harmful for physical health.

The same series of tests were performed for retirement taken alone with controls, and then all taken with the interaction factors for the outcome measure of life satisfaction. Retirement's hypothesized negative effects upon men's life satisfaction, either independently or in interaction with specific factors, were not substantiated by the analysis.

The same series of tests were performed for retirement taken alone with controls, and then all taken with the same interaction factors for the outcome measure of physical health satisfaction. Retirement's hypothesized negative effects upon physical health satisfaction were not supported when retirement was tested independently. However, when taken in the context of the income and education interactive terms, retirement becomes a singular positive predictor for *good* physical health satisfaction. Moreover, when retirement was tested in interaction with the Retirement x Income (T1) term, that interaction term itself became a significant predictor for positive physical health satisfaction for low-income men. These results reject the hypothesis that retirement is *harmful* for physical health satisfaction.

A notable aspect of this significant interaction deals with low-income older *workers* (the comparison group). While workers of all income levels except the highest have negative physical health satis-faction levels, low-income workers have very low physical health satisfaction when compared to low-income retirees. These men have been working under conditions of low income. Their feelings of life satisfaction have suffered throughout this period of employ-ment, and now that they are *older* workers, they may have danger-ously low levels of life satisfaction. They probably have also devel-oped poor physical health while working.

The situation of sickly low-income workers calls for the careful attention of mental health professionals. Again, it is important to look at older worker attitudes about their health and lives. Perhaps these men feel that health matters are *outside* their control. For economic reasons they must continue to work, despite the fact that they are in poor physical health. Work itself contributed to their poor health. They probably have the benefit of company-paid health insurance and could attend to health problems as they occur. However, as is usually the case in American society, medical care is not sought (nor paid for by insurance) as a preventive measure, but only when a health problem has developed. Physical damage to the human body has been done. These men are older men; convalescence is long and may not be totally successful. Moreover, these men must return to the workplace in all probability.

It seems that in the total picture of their situation as sickly, low-income workers, the social benefits of work are outweighed by the negative physical health consequences of work. Work is a major component of their lives. Resultant life dissatisfaction is probably the first poor mental health symptom. The likelihood of this poor life satisfaction spilling over and negatively affecting physical health satisfaction is great, as the results with this sample of older workers imply. Thus, it is reasonable to speculate that they then developed poor mental health (measured by poor physical health satisfaction). Again, this finding points to the fact that *retirement* seems to be beneficial for low-income men's mental health.

Sometimes researchers who do secondary analyses do not have sufficient information from their studies to speculate about the direction of the effects between relevant factors in their hypotheses. In this case, the triad of physical health status, life satisfaction, and physical health satisfaction is the issue for low-income workers. With these low-income workers, it is important to determine what came first, poor physical health or low life satisfaction. Then, a progressive pattern of development can be etched to determine the causal route that culminates in poor physical health satisfaction. This inquiry holds potential for future primary research.

Likewise, future research should look more closely at the relationship between work attitudes and retirement attitudes among low-income older workers. The qualitative differences between work and retirement attitudes may be very wide. As discussed in the previous chapter, work attitudes may be extremely negative, and the time for retirement is anxiously awaited as a relief from the hardships of work. Is that wide difference in attitudes itself problematic? How does that attitudinal imbalance affect: (1) their physical and mental health as older workers, and (2) their physical and mental health as retirees? This current research suggests that physical and mental health should improve markedly for low-income older workers once they retire. Accurate and tested causal links must be established by research if the physical and mental health of older workers is to be better safeguarded by health professionals.

The current physical health of retirees is positively affected only by their prior physical health. What is noteworthy is the fact that the retirement experience for men (even with the death of their spouse/ significant other) has no significant *harmful effects* whatsoever on physical health. Therefore, declining physical health *cannot* be made attributable to retirement.

The mental health of retirees seems to have been undamaged by retirement (or death of a spouse/significant other, in some cases). Thus, it could be that many retirees have been able to *cope* with retirement (*and* death of a spouse/significant other) because they have already constructed the necessary supportive resources in their lives. Adjustment to their post-retirement life is successfully made because physical health, psychological, social, and/or economic resources are available to them, perceived by them to be available when needed, and used when needed. These men have satisfactorily replaced work-related friendships and activities with other meaningful relationships and activities.

Perhaps retired men who also lost wives or significant others have been able to adjust to their losses without losing their good mental health. These life events may not be as stressful as previously believed by some researchers, at least with regard to the measures of mental health that this study assesses. It would be interesting to do additional analyses with the same sample but now controlling for prior mental health. If the results are different from this current study's, one could then deduce that good mental health had been developed in these men while they were working and married, and served them well through retirement and death of a spouse/significant other. One could also speculate that these men were in particularly positive social circumstances as younger adults.

This research suggests that retirement can have beneficial consequences for many men. The "aging/increasing life satisfaction" relationship can spill over and increase physical health satisfaction for some retired men. Thus, most men in this study who retire (and grow older) seem to be able to reconcile life's differences and maintain or increase their life satisfaction, while also accepting their physical finiteness and frailties with a satisfactory outlook. The American retirement system has functioned well for the majority of retired men in this four year study. Physical health and life satisfaction are not negatively affected by retirement. Physical health satisfaction is positive for retirees but negative for those low-income men not yet retired. In the *four year* time frame of this study in which the effects of retirement are examined, physical health and mental health are good. This implies minimal or satisfactory interaction with the American health care system.

This study's implication that retirement can be beneficial for some men serves to question literature that asserts that retirement is harmful. This study's theoretical model holds that retirement and death of a spouse/ significant other are *harmful* for men's physical and mental health (Holmes and Rahe, 1967; Cutrona et al., 1986; Cassel, 1976a; Cassel, 1976b; Atchley, 1976; Haynes et al., 1977). Much of past research is also generous with evidence that these life events produce debilitating stress that is harmful for self-esteem and disruptive of social systems (Preston and Mansfield, 1984; Lin et al., 1979; Linn, 1986).

However, an examination of the data presented in this current study finds that retirement and\or death of a spouse/significant other are *not* debilitating to men's physical or mental health. Retirement can have *beneficial* consequences for low income men's physical health satisfaction. This finding calls for a re-evaluation of stressful life event theory when scientists consider retirement. It may be that the stress of retirement can be productively used to help engage or create a person's social networks and raise self-esteem.

Despite this optimistic picture, one must also examine this life situation with a longer range perspective that looks beyond the limited four year time frame of this study. With a greater time frame for more information gathering, significant research findings are more likely to arise and to be put to maximum use. (Retirement, per se, may not be implicated in these new findings.) This larger view encompasses a greater reality but tends to be more negative. Retired men are at growing risk for physical and mental health problems because of the natural *aging* process that extends beyond retirement. Moreover, men die earlier than women.

National data indicate that all populations of older men are bound to increase (Russell, 1981). Most older men (as workers or retirees), thus, sometime in their lives become needy of *comprehensive* health care that attends to both physical and mental health. They will most assuredly be forced to seek services from the dominant medical system in America. These services may prove to be far from comprehensive. Low-income older workers that have low physical health satisfaction are particularly at risk. Research such as this must be used as problem-solving information by health care professionals who render services to low-income working men.

The final chapter will present policy and programmatic recommendations for comprehensive and improved health care for the older adult population in light of their specific needs and the growing numbers of elderly persons (especially those 85 years old and older). The chapter will first discuss relevant characteristics of the unsatisfactory physician-dominated American health care delivery system, present-day community-based health care programs for older adults in America, and ways in which community programs are geared toward primary, secondary, and tertiary health care for older adults. These programs promote healthful lifestyles that allow older adults to function at their maximum levels. Second, the role of the social worker as policy-maker and practitioner in these pursuits is given particular attention because historically the social work profession has concerned itself with populations at risk, such as the elderly. The aging retired male, in these times, has come to be seen as particularly vulnerable to the stresses of life and health problems inherent in his last cycle of life. Third, the present and future roles of health care policy for older Americans (with comparisons to national health policies in select countries), the role of research in older adult health care, and rationales for future health care are discussed.

Chapter VIII

## POLICY AND PROGRAMMATIC
## RECOMMENDATIONS FOR COMPREHENSIVE
## OLDER ADULT HEALTH CARE

Current American health care relies primarily on physician-dominated perspectives for treatment and care that are *not* comprehensive. (Physician-related treatment is administered mainly in institutions, with little reliance on community-based facilities.) Older retired men face difficulties when they seek physical and mental health care from this established system.

### Why the Current Health Care System
### for Older Men Must Change

Adults over 65 represent only 11 percent of the population in America, yet they are responsible for 25 percent to 30 percent of health care expenditures (Ford, 1981; Branch et al., 1984). They spend 11 percent of their income on health care and account for 22 percent of physician charges, 28 percent of hospital costs, and 89 percent of skilled nursing facility costs (Ford, 1981). Older people identified poor health and the cost of health care as more serious concerns than retirement or death of a spouse/significant other in a 1981 National Council on Aging survey by Lou Harris (Jacobs and Abbott, 1983).

The likelihood of the above situation remaining the same or worsening in the future is very great if American health care for older adults is not improved in the near future. As discussed in Chapter I, the retired population, a large subcategory of all older adults, is increasing in number with *great* speed. This growth is causing concern because the American health care system is not prepared to handle the likely health care needs of this population. Despite the fact that the medical system has made great advances in many aspects of health care for all populations in recent decades, excessive medical care may harm patients. Moreover, *chronic illnesses and many stress-related disorders*, which tend to strike the elderly, still have no cures and require psychosocial as well as medical intervention.

Moreover, the dominant medical system determines how older people use medical care. Current medical expectations encourage older people to depend only upon the system itself for health maintenance and do not foster self-reliance (Mechanic, 1979; Dychtwald, 1983). Such dependence is remunerative for the system, and therefore many powerful professionals with interests entrenched in the status quo have resisted attempts to alter the system. However, concerned and capable professionals including social workers and psychologists must *modify* the system if the health care needs of the elderly are to be comprehensively addressed and satisfied.

The medical system defines acute care as the primary avenue for all health care, despite the fact that many retired, older men do not always need acute medical care. Often, hospitalization *is not* needed for chronic conditions or stress-related illnesses when they strike older men. In fact, Monnig (1980) reports that the elderly participants in his study infrequently cite the need for high-technology medical care; they prefer to remain independent and rely on therapeutic self-care for improvements in health.

Consequently, high-technology and hospital-centered interventions are of limited use many times. Standard medical care (physicians, drugs and hospitals) provides for only 10 percent of an individual's health needs (Preston and Mansfield, 1984). The remaining 90 percent of health needs respond to psychosocial factors in retired men's lives such as social conditions, personal adjustment and coping abilities, and stress levels, over which physicians have little control or expertise, if any (Health Maintenance and Health Promotion, 1981; Health Promotion for Older Persons, 1982; Cluff, 1983; Green, 1985).

It is not surprising that Lorig et al., (1984) find that self-care leads to reduced physician visits. The literature makes two observations about self-care behaviors: 1) the elderly themselves are able to distinguish between their important and non-important symptoms, and 2) the health complaints of the elderly are, by and large, valid (Eckstein, 1976; Shanas and Maddox, 1983).

While older men certainly have numerous acute health episodes, chronic conditions are more pervasive. Stress-related illnesses are common. Eighty-five percent of adults 65 years and older suffer from "afflictions of civilization": chronic, degenerative, largely in-curable diseases (Ford, 1981; Pelletier, 1983; Rabin, 1984). These diseases are determined by lifestyle, social environment, physical environment, and are possible to prevent, postpone, or ameliorate to an extent (Preston and Mansfield, 1984). In fact, healthful patterns of eating, drinking, exercising, drug and tobacco use, and reduction of stress can minimize the likelihood of illness (Sorenson and Ford, 1981; Wells, 1982; Krehl, 1983; Pelletier, 1983). This alternative disease concept is particularly relevant to older men who experience stressful life events such as retirement or death of a spouse/signifi-cant other.

Therefore, the clinical protocol of the current medical care system, in which physicians are assertive technicians and elderly patients are passive consumers, is not the most efficacious approach (Jacobs and Abbott, 1983). Proper management of older adults' stess-related illnesses dictates that long-term psychosocial inter-ventions are often necessary despite medical interventions (Schrock, 1980; Whitbourne and Sperneck, 1981; Dychtwald, 1983). To serve the medical needs of retirees without regard to psychosocial needs is half-baked health care.

Research reveals a decline in physician visits by people 75 years and older and a "reluctance for extravagant physician use" by many elderly people even when they have unlimited access to physicians (Eckstein, 1976; Barney and Neukom, 1977). Many health care professionals hold unfavorable attitudes toward care of older adults as do many Americans (German, 1975). Just as important, the traditional hospital approach of treating a patient after the disease has developed is also costly, especially for older retired people whose income may be reduced. However, it is noteworthy that a portion of all older adults—regardless of income—choose *not* to seek assis-tance from the formal medical system. Major reasons are psycho-logical: fear and lack of trust in physicians (Shanas and Maddox, 1983).

Stults (1984), a physician, estimates that considerable time and expense would be required to initiate comprehensive programs for the elderly in all settings. The American medical system has never been geared to comprehensive health care. He cites these obstacles: physicians visiting patients irregularly, physicians having negative attitudes toward the elderly, elderly persons reporting illnesses late, and the financing of health care being heavily geared toward acute health care. Thus, much of the responsibility for planning, designing, and implementing preventive health programs will be assumed by non-physician professionals such as social workers, psychologists, nurses, educators, and therapists.

## Programs With a
## "Wellness" Perspective

Luckily, some hospitals have programs with a "wellness" perspective. These programs integrate psychosocial factors into hospital service-delivery and can assist individuals such as retired men to achieve good physical and mental health. Such factors include allowing patients to feel self-reliant and "in control" by patient participation in decision-making, and group therapeutic methods (Peck et al., 1983).

However, community health programs still are more able than hospitals to incorporate a more comprehensive and continuous holistic perspective into their service-delivery methods. The holistic perspective of health promotion programs meets specific needs of retired men by integrating characteristics of body, mind and spirit; social, economic, political, and environmental factors; consumer responsibility; and an equitable structure of power between service providers and recipients into its operation (Dychtwald, 1983).

Many community health programs are intent on using balanced relationships of factors such as those mentioned above to reach outcomes of good health for older men. Such programs can be beneficial for retirees with poor physical health and/or low life satisfaction. The basic philosophical premise of health promotion programs is a need to motivate all older adults to become better informed and assume more responsibility for their own health. Community-based health care and wellness programs for older adults provide continuity of care, and opportunities for self-care before and after health status changes in their delivery of professional health care services. This provision of services, thus, fosters, client self-determination and self-control, and improves psychological as well as physical well-being (Lederman et al., 1983; Lurie and Shulman, 1983; Crump and Lewis, 1985).

Health education and pre-retirement training programs can include information about nutrition, self-care, disease and disability prevention, and physical fitness. These health care programs reflect new societal circumstances, multidisciplinary team implementation, and effective educational and self-care approaches (Butler et al., 1979; Shamansky and Hamilton, 1979; Hickey, 1980; Lederman et al., 1980; Warner-Reitz and Mettler, 1983; Johnson, 1984; Longe and Wolf, 1985). Programs need to be continually reformulated if American society is to avoid tragic consequences because of the threat the health care system poses to retirees' income and well-being, not to mention the national budget.

## Priority Objectives to Improve Primary, Secondary, and Tertiary Preventive Service-Delivery for Older Adults

The examination of the health status of retired, older adults in Chapter II reveals a spectrum of ailments ranging from acute diseases to chronic ailments (Shanas, 1980). While the task of primary prevention is integral to health promotion programs for older adults, primary preventive techniques may not be appropriate in many cases because of the chronic and stress-related natures of many of their health problems. Health promotion must, therefore, become more comprehensive for elderly persons and also offer secondary and tertiary health care.

It is important to understand the distinctions among these types of health care. Primary prevention deals with the disease-free state. Its goal is to avert disease, injuries or defects. Secondary prevention deals with the symptom phase. Its goal is to detect disease early. Tertiary prevention deals with the developed disease and its aftermath. Its goals involve prevention of the progression of disability, and the improvement of functioning and quality of life (Rabin, 1984).

The tailoring of preventive health care to the unique needs of retired men represents a top priority objective for older adult health care programs. With a main objective of primary care, health promotion programs and policies are currently emphasizing primary and secondary prevention and excluding tertiary prevention (Rabin, 1984). However, because of the nature of many of the elderly's health problems, these three types of prevention may be called for with the same person for a combination of problems.

The general process of prevention involves identifying health risks in an older man's life plus instilling motivation in him to minimize the risks. To facilitate risk self-identification among clients, Crump and Lewis (1985) suggest that the established medical care system be used as a vehicle to provide more preventive information to the consumer. Assessment tools must be used that will identify the elderly at risk before illness. For instance, as the results of the present study suggest, certain numbers of all retired men develop illnesses while working. Alarmingly, high-income retirees also have poor health satisfaction and this is an indicator of poor mental health. The proper point for preventive intervention for *future* retirees would be, therefore, while they are still in the workplace. Moreover, the study also shows that the older men who are still working, have poor mental health shown by low levels of physical health satisfaction, conceivably because their physical health is bad. This, too, indicates that working life is a good time for preventive care for physical and mental health.

Preventive interventions for older men can result in positive behavior change (unhealthful habits become health oriented), a decrease in morbidity, and a postponement of death (Rakowski, 1985). Prior medical examinations, health education, proper nutrition, or exercise can *delay* or *prevent* onset of physical health problems (Hickey, 1980). However, this self-prevention process is commonly complicated by the difficulty older adults may have in recognizing the early signs of disease. In addition, many older adults do not seek any sort of care until the condition has developed.

With the goal of meaningful health care for older adults, Butler et al. (1979) say that group dynamics, behavior modification, and social support ought to be used in health education programs. Community programs facilitate goals of good health care through a variety of well-tested techniques. For instance, group interventions with retired, elderly persons may facilitate participant management of their environment and engender feelings of self-efficacy among them (Nickoley-Colquitt, 1981). This is particularly important for retired men because some of them may not have adjusted very well to retirement. They are not able to compensate for the social and psychological support systems that existed at work.

In medical self-help groups, persons with similar health problems meet to share information, experiences, coping mechanisms and to assist each other in tertiary prevention. Social support systems are thus created that ease life for the afflicted, and may be useful for those high-income retirees who have relatively low physical health satisfaction.

Community-based programs of these types are still in early stages of development. Anderson (1981) calls for multiservice measures to combat lifestyle diseases through a continuum of preventive practices involving motivation, education, exercise, and nutrition. Dychtwald's (1983) theoretical perspective builds on Anderson's. Because so much of the chronic disease process is noninfectious and modifiable, Dychtwald is primarily interested in instilling and eliciting self-responsibility and health vitality in older people. These last two perspectives extend health prevention beyond the traditional medical model into the psychosocial model.

Despite these progressive theoretical models, tertiary prevention—or rehabilitation—today remains, in practice, an underdeveloped area that has received relatively little professional effort. Extensive and coordinated community services are lacking. Rehabilitation care providers are few and generally work in hospitals, not in community-based facilities (Health Maintenance and Health Promotion, 1981). The Federal handling of rehabilitative care has been equally unimpressive. Now placed in the Department of Education, the Rehabilitation Services Administration (RSA) does not provide necessary comprehensive services to older adults. The RSA should be reassigned to Health and Human Services to better allow for necessary professional linkages (Health Maintenance and Health Promotion, 1981).

Tertiary prevention must receive higher priority. Methods of service-delivery must be redeveloped in the traditional medical system *and* in community programs if the diverse population of retired men (and older workers) are going to be provided with appropriate care to allow maximum functioning. To facilitate this redevelopment, Hickey (1980) emphasizes that long-term care must be redefined to include more than institutionalization. Tertiary care should also be interpreted as beginning in the family environment and should include the coping behaviors of the chronically ill older patient (Hickey, 1980). As a result of this redevelopment, when retired men become less physically and/or mentally independent, they would be able to turn to the community for health and social services, and preserve their independence rather than enter an institution.

## The Social Work Role in Health
## Care for the Older Adult

Because of an underdeveloped geriatric medical subspecialty in this country, comprehensive physical and mental health care services are not readily available to all older adults.  However, social workers, psychologists and other allied health care professionals are primary service providers in effective medical and psychosocial health care programs that tend to be more comprehensive and satisfactory.  They contact elderly patients more frequently than attending physicians, in many cases.  Therefore, they may more strongly influence patients' health behavior because of the potential for exchanging meaningful information.  In the case of older retired men who are socially isolated, information may take the forms of referrals to expand social networks, of psychosocial counseling aimed at improving mental health, or of alternatives for health services.

Being multiskilled professionals, social workers have numerous critical roles in the delivery of these services, as evidenced by extensive research and publications (Bloom, 1980). [Please see the Appendix for a listing of examples of hospital and community programs that use social workers as members of the health team.] Epstein (1980) sees social workers as program planners in health care who analyze problems from a psychosocial perspective and select options based on social work values.  Social workers also design and evaluate programs.  In all these tasks, however, the social work role is guided by current health care policy and related research.

Social work services offered in all health care settings reflect two fundamental characteristics of the social work profession: flexibility and adaptation.  These characteristics exist within a framework of specialized skills in a variety of job environments. Social work training is specialized enough to prepare workers for intervention with populations at risk in a particular setting, such as retired elderly men in a hospital or other institution. In such a setting, the social worker works with these men because they may have difficulty adjusting to their social situations because of poor chronic or stress-related illnesses. The social worker establishes relationships with these men, holistically assesses their situations, makes appropriate referrals, and, perhaps, begins case management with them.

However, rigorous social work training also emphasizes breadth of knowledge that allows the same workers to function professionally in a community setting such as a Senior Citizens Center or a Community Mental Health Center where the workers are likely to treat retired men. The settings have characteristics distinct from institutions. In a community setting, social workers usually influence older adult participants even more because of more professional autonomy, and a consequent more personal and consistent social context. Here, a social worker incorporates the functions of a hospital social worker with the design, administration, or implementation of projects that can range from medical screenings, to nutrition programs, to social activities.

Social work theories form the conceptual framework of many innovative health promotion and prevention programs for older adults (Health Promotion for Older Persons: Group Program Models, 1982; Butler et al., 1979; Sorenson and Ford, 1981; Lurie and Shulman, 1983; Dana, 1983; Barbaro and Noyes, 1984; Green, 1985). The social work profession emphasizes an interdisciplinary teamwork approach for health care service delivery that also develops client self-determination and personal responsibility. Social workers have also been developers and proponents of group theory and group work in their mission to preserve patient rights while helping the patient to improve health.

Research has shown that the most helpful way to improve the habits and thought patterns of older adults is not necessarily through medical intervention but through group activities (Nickoley-Colquitt, 1981). Groups represent the most effective intervention to assist in the various socialization processes necessary to achieve program goals. Thus, groups act to make new social ties available. This is especially important for older retired men who may need self-esteem boosters and increased social networks.

Adult education helps group members achieve individual goals for personal growth. Except for social workers trained in group therapy, few professionals in the health care setting have received any training on how to teach adults (Apgar and Coplon, 1985). Likewise, other professionals on the team (except for psychologists and, to a lesser degree, psychiatrists) are not trained or responsible for social aspects of health. In the case of this study's findings, social workers running pre-retirement training sessions should more actively address aging and health issues, and relate them to mental health because results show health satisfaction to decrease with the retired sample as income increased.

Northen (1983) suggests social work groups be used in health care settings to influence client change regarding those psychosocial factors that "predispose, precipitate, or perpetuate" illness. In a similar vein, Hickey (1980) writes of the need for psychosocial interventions as older adults' health care dependencies increase. He advocates for social worker-run teams and groups as effective therapeutic measures. For instance, social workers frequently use their group work knowledge in fitness programs with older adults that could be particularly therapeutic for retirees in poor health. These programs satisfy their physical, psychological, as well as social needs.

Programs such as these, according to Dana (1983) are based on continuity in primary, secondary, and tertiary preventive care. Client motivation is the key element and she thus advocates that social workers:

1.  focus on changing behavior in the environment to eradicate those conditions associated with high morbidity and mortality,

2.  help people to change adverse behavior before the onset of illness, assist the community in the development and maintenance of support systems, advocate for insurance coverage for health education and support services,

3.  help the identified sick achieve and maintain the highest level of social and physical functioning possible.

This current study illuminates factors concerning retired men *and* older workers that can be applied to Dana's theoretical framework. In point #1 above, social workers must investigate the work environment as a key site for preventive intervention and must strive to reach health care goals according to the time-line in point #2: *before* retirement (while still at the worksite). Lastly, sickly retirees can be maintained at home in reasonable good health through community health programs, as stated in point #3.

For men who retire because of poor health, motivation must develop in their pre-retirement years. Sickly retired men require sensitive motivation that utilizes social worker skills, resources, and knowledge as ingredients for patient development. These ingredients may consist of needs assessments, case management, referrals, and education. The social worker can act as an important facilitator to achieve the positive behavior change necessary for the improved well-being of retired men whose resources may be few.

Furthermore, social workers can play influential roles in establishing a viable basis for preventive health care services for older adults discussed in the earlier part of this chapter, as they did in the 1920s for maternal-child preventive health care (Siefert, 1983). In the 1920s, social workers secured funds, planned, designed and implemented many badly needed preventive services. Today, social workers create similar crisis-oriented programs for many types of social problems but also evaluate programming and engage in research. In doing so, social workers act as proponents of a "call to action" among health professionals to improve health care for older adults. This "action" is part of the social work mission.

However, there must also be political motivation, in addition to health-care-driven goals, if there are going to be major improvements in the American health care system. As advocates for older persons' rights and necessary health policy changes, social workers further demonstrate their crucial roles as political liaisons. Social workers must ultimately act as the gatekeeper for the clients' rights while they also function as middle men for communications among service providers, patients, policy-makers, and politicians.

## Policy and Research Roles: the Present and the Future

### The Roles of Policy

**Comparative World Health Policy.** The research by Checkoway and Betancourt (1989) illustrates that nations of different sociopolitical persuasions from America are dealing with their elderly health care situation in more humane and effective ways. America can learn from the examples of Canada, Israel, England, Scotland, West Germany, Denmark, and Sweden. These nations have fashioned viable partnerships between their federal/ municipal governments and community agencies with the one objective of improving the health of the elderly. These collaborations have generated and sustained successful programs that have become integral parts of their societies (Checkoway and Betancourt, 1989). Factors aiding the positive momentum of these programs are a national commitment, skillful design and implementation of programs, sufficient funding, and the lack of social stigma attached to participation in welfare programs among the elderly.

Although these programs are "government welfare programs" by definition, these societies have deemed citizen participation in these programs as an inalienable right of the populace with no inherent shame. These nations have confronted the physical and mental health problems of their older citizens with clear purposes and integrity, and the results are progressive and comprehensive. Health care for older adults in these nations is accessible, affordable, and competent.

However, the situation in the United States is quite different. First, American society has stigmatized the receipt of government welfare as a desperate shame. Second, despite the escalating population of older persons, which has been discernible since before World War II, American society has neglected to prepare itself for this population shift. At best, American society is dealing with this problem belatedly and begrudgingly. Community-based social service programming for older people has existed since the 1950s, but has often been short-lived because of constrained and time-limited funding and the perennial "welfare stigma". Thus, today federal and state commitment to older adult health care research and programming is haphazard and unsatisfactory for elderly patients.

**American Health Care Policy**. Medicaid and Medicare, as proposed solutions to the American health care dilemma, have proven in contemporary times to be less than fulfilling, as mentioned in Chapter I. For instance, since their inception, there has been an overdevelopment of nursing homes at the expense of badly needed social services for the elderly (Jacobs and Abbott, 1983). Russell

(1981) predicts an *increase* in the institutionalization of older adults through 2050 if our current system remains unchanged.

The current structure of Medicaid and Medicare effectively *blocks* potential use of *preventive* medical services. Medicaid covers the bulk of long-term care, but the individual must be at the poverty level or below to qualify. Medicaid also provides no incentive for preventive care. It does not encourage the necessary linkages between medical services and social services, and makes limited provisions for home health care (TenHoor, 1982). Medicare has been estimated to cover only about 40 percent of the total health care costs of older adults, and provides insurance coverage for *only* hospital-related, physician-prescribed treatment (Ford, 1981). Serious chronic conditions which may be treatable at one's home by a community agency do not qualify, despite the fact that home treatment is preferred over hospital treatment by many older adults. Moreover, it is a proven cost-effective alternative.

In a recent attempt to control costs, hospitals have introduced the mechanism known as diagnostic referral groups (DRGs). This new policy has, perhaps, contained some expenses but to the consternation of the American Medical Association (Health Care for Elders, 1984). However, the American Medical Association-dominated medical system is nonetheless responsible for patient neglect. Elderly patients are frequently being discharged prematurely because their stay at a hospital is time-limited and pre-arranged. Elderly patients do not represent cost-effective endeavors for the system or physicians in our classical American supply-side economic model (Health Care for Elders, 1984).

What then is an effective way to control the unrelentingly expanding costs of American health care?

There is little evidence that *physician self-regulation* reduces costs (Ford, 1981). Alarmingly, a growing number of physicians are regulating patient intake and are no longer accepting Medicare because of reimbursements they consider insufficient (Jacobs and Abbott, 1983). Therefore, despite projections of an overabundance of physicians, the future of health care remains a strong concern for older adults because physicians have proven to be less concerned with their roles as "helping professionals" and more concerned with material work benefits. Moreover, the only cost-effective targets for purposive cost controls are physicians' fees for services—both direct services and physician-referred services.

Green (1985) argues that although many physicians are skilled technicians and medical technology has become more complex, there is little increase in the success rate of patient care and cure. She cites the present death rate in America as remaining close to what it was at the turn of the century. Wells (1981) states that life expectancy has not increased significantly since 1962, despite massive health care expenditures by the system and consumers.

Expectedly, developments in medical technology have increased the costs of a typical medical encounter. Ironically, *more* but different facilities, and *more* skilled personnel are needed to fill the widening *gap* between health care services available in the current system and elderly patients actual needs. This does not bode well for future efforts at health care cost containment when future trands in care are based on the current self-endorsing medical care system.

It is evident that the U.S. health care system must accurately reconceptualize all facets of aging because this phenomenon is reaching mammoth proportions. This widened view must include more sensitive and holistic perspectives of care, and greater use of psychosocial dynamics. New attempts at cost controls are factors which must be incorporated into new health care policy if this policy is to contribute to improved services for older adults (Schrock, 1980; Whitbourne and Spernack, 1981; Dychtwald, 1983; Green, 1985).

**Policy "Gaps."** The term "gaps" refers to the fact that there is no solution in the current scheme of health care systems policy to solve a current health or social problem, or a predicted one. A problem may have been identified, and interventions may have been implemented with a modicum of success, but because of political or bureaucratic hindrances, or funding constraints, these services are not readily available or accessible to the relevant populations. The problem, thus, may not be adequately addressed any longer.

Gaps particularly affect retired, older adults whose income is too high to qualify for Medicaid yet too low to be able to purchase additional health insurance. Older persons of all incomes with chronic illnesses, in particular, are overlooked. Ford (1981) points to the increasing prevalence of chronic illnesses *since* Medicare's legislation. Medicare has not positively affected overall health status, nor has it reduced the number of persons who are homebound or bedfast

(Shanas, 1980; Spring, 1981). Older adults who need services of the American health care service delivery system face serious impediments because of these gaps.

Some of this study's results may stem from some of American health policy's insufficiencies. First, one result (see Figure 2) shows that high-income retirees tend to have poorer physical health satisfaction than their low-income counterparts. One may speculate that these high-income men have poor physical health and that some of their problems are chronic. Perhaps these health problems originated during pre-retirement years and could have been prevented. However, the early section of this final chapter argues that the American medical system is *not* geared to prevention. So now that men are retired, they *cannot* depend on Medicare to pay for in-home health services or community health services. They must first go to an approved institution and see a physican under the auspices of Medicare. Then, they would be eligible only for physician-referred home services.

They may be forced to purchase private health insurance, or pay cash for services (and, perhaps, risk spend-down of financial resources). With sufficient spend-down, these persons may qualify for Medicaid—a consequence of reduced socioeconomic status. However, all of these options may be bad for mental health.

Second, older *workers* in the study are faced with similar hardships. Their mental health is not good for the most part, except for high-income workers as the significant interaction in Figure 2 shows. They are consumers in a society in which its health care system does not value prevention or economy. They participate in job environments that may be harmful to their physical health. Moreover, when workers become eligible for Medicare (some already are), Medicare will *not* cover non-institutional care that is not medically acute and physician driven. In-home prevention and health maintenance to allow continued workforce participation becomes nearly impossible to achieve.

In the realm of preventive programs, these impediments would be minimized by policy directed at redesigning social and economic environments to reduce risks for older adults. Community agencies and health care services must be coordinated and expanded to achieve full preventive goals. Multiservice agencies are providing some preventive services with some success; however, agencies of this sort are not widespread or well funded across the United States. Preventive programs must be located in diverse geographical settings to reach the different older adult populations at risk and should include pre-retirement training programs, life care communities, hospital and medical school-related programs, government programs, and private sector programs (Dychtwald, 1978; Anderson, 1981; Sorenson, 1981; Health Promotion for Older Persons, 1982; Lederman et al., 1983; Peck et al., 1983; Simmons et al., 1983; Barbaro and Noyes, 1984; Longe and Wolf, 1984; Lorig et al., 1984). Policy-makers must exhibit improved commitment and integrity in their mission if they are to be successful at improving health care for the elderly.

## The Roles of Research

Interest in research about older adult health care can be traced to the 1950s, but its growth roughly coincides with the early years of Medicare, a decade later. Research on community-based health care for the elderly is currently in a relatively underdeveloped stage, especially when compared to other areas of scientific inquiry (Dana, 1983). When an observer takes into consideration the fact that research concerning allied health professions and non-medical interventions has not been given high priority in the Federal budget or in the American medical system, one begins to understand reasons for the delayed growth of health care research for older adults and the limited health care gains (Dana, 1983).

The growth of older adult populations well into the third decade of the next century *must* result in health care professionals looking to broader focused research concerning health care needs if these professionals are going to advocate for new policy. Present data points to a variety of issues that will be of vital concern to researchers: increasing health care and insurance costs, increasing policy conflicts, chronic health problems, the shortcomings of our present health care delivery system, alternative health care services, and the changing definitions and meanings of the aging process.

These issues are serious and *remain* unresolved despite the sophistication of medical technology. Gerontological research on community-based health care must expand to include relevant health care for the diverse older population if health care for the elderly is to be improved. This sort of productive research stimulates the establishment of effective health care policy and programs.

Research is also needed to give a sound base to professional education about health care for the elderly. Knowledge is lacking about the functional determinants of older adults' health, functional outcomes of services administered to them, and the preventive and maintenance behaviors that are of *greatest benefit* to them (Committee on the Aging Society, 1985). Information about active life expectancy, which measures independence in activities of daily living, and activity theory, which holds that activity is positively associated with good mental health, are necessary elements of a practical knowledge base, but are currently missing from many new health policy formulations.

Gaps in knowledge can be created by a lack of true multidisciplinary efforts on the part of the service-delivery health care team to attend to all factors in older men's lives. In the lopsided American health care system, where the medical discipline dominates the "team," team efforts may be insufficient and incomplete. Important patient issues may go unattended, and often they are psychosocial in nature, *not* medical. These gaps of knowledge are preventing policy-makers from making judicious decisions regarding proper delivery of health care services to retired, older men.

Researchers can fill in these gaps by developing information about the biological, psychological, social, and environmental factors involved in health care. As this study shows, these factors are affected by the retirement and post-retirement experiences of older men, as well as worklife experiences of the older worker. Research knowledge, such as is presented here, acts as a stimulus for new policy. Policy-making is an attempt to create a synthesis of resources, goals, values, and motivation (Hetherington and Calderone, 1985). New policy would ultimately translate into improving the service goals of programs, as well as restructuring entitlement programs to more effectively address population needs. Researchers and policy-makers must interact for effective programming to develop. Current health care research, which often breeds health care programs that are insufficient and not comprehensive, represents only weak attempts to reach solutions.

## Rationales for Future Research in Health Care

Rationales for expanded awarenesses and new emphases in the health care system are often products factors that seem functionally unrelated in American society. These factors consist of increased medical care costs, the continued prevalence of chronic conditions, and, studies that link health and behavior (Mechanic, 1979). However, relationships among the biomedical, social, environmental, economic and psychological spheres of human life are indisputable, as this current research concerning retirement and health has shown.

This research will undoubtedly serve to educate professionals and students, and will afford them new understandings of older adult health care needs. However, while some elder health care needs are being treated, others remain unresolved. Moreover, new ones arise as society changes. This research exemplifies that men who have retired for poor health, and low-income older workers may very well be *at risk* for deteriorating physical and mental health, yet are *overlooked* by the "system." The functions of health promotion programs in the near future will be to more adequately meet the health care needs of these older adults that the present system is neglecting.

Health promotion programs are often hospital-based, yet there are also successful examples of community-based ones (see page 149). This research suggests two new foci for health promotion programs. The first focus will be to work holistically with older workers and retirees in and out of institutions in efforts to achieve disease prevention, health promotion, rehabilitation, and health maintenance. In this way, older persons can prevent or minimize institutionalization, preserve functional independence, and reduce social isolation (Barbaro and Noyes, 1984). The second focus would be to contain or lower health care costs by reducing ultimately the number of contacts with physicians and/or hospitals, and engaging the elderly in alternative community health care. With widespread networks of community- and hospital-based health promotion programs, lifestyles will become more healthful as self-responsibility increases, and costs to the consumer and the system will decrease (Ford, 1981).

These successful programs must be regularly evaluated to create a recipe for effective programming. Evaluating the effectiveness of current programs is critical to allow policy-makers and planners to redesign efforts to meet the health care needs of the growing population of retirees. The process of program accountability would measure mortality, morbidity, quality of life, behavior change, and productivity of the consumers, and the cost-effectiveness of the operating system.

Basically, policies and programs have professional and moral obligations to present a balanced picture of expected benefits, availability of resources to meet such goals, and existing limitations (Rakowski, 1985). Because the American health care system is not currently meetying this need satisfactorily, two final suggestions are put forth to improve the situation. First, the diversity of health care professionals in America, economists, *and* lawmakers must *together* re-evaluate America's national priorities concerning the health of older adults. The physical and mental health of retired men and those men nearing retirement must be examined seriously, and community health services must be expanded and made accessible to all older adults.

Second, research must now focus on tapping heretofore unexamined data. This study is a good example of how useful information can be gathered when one studies a subgroup of a larger population for specific purposes, in this case retired men, and physical and mental health. The current research was a secondary analysis, and did not provide sufficiently detailed data for the resultant depth of the inquiry. Speculations had to be made about the results. However, the literature review and the research design of this study offer solid foundation for continued inquiry into this matter.

A similar design could be followed in new primary research with other *subgroups and issues* to determine retirement's effects, for example, retired *women*; the various ethnic groups of retired men and women; those persons, in particular, who retired prematurely because of poor physical health; the relationship of retirement to changing patterns of alcohol consumption; and the plights of older (low-income) workers. This future research must work with data that is relevant and powerful. Only then will improvements in health care for all American older adults be forthcoming.

# APPENDICES

Appendix A

# A SAMPLE OF HEALTH PROMOTION
# PROGRAMS IN AMERICA

The following are examples of health promotion programs in which the social work profession has been a major partner:

1. *Wallingford Wellness Project, Seattle, WA*: The program design, purpose and service-delivery is based on social work principles: improve health through education and behavior change. The project is affiliated with University of Washington School of Social Work.

2. *Growing Younger Program, Boise, ID:* The program's emphasis on self-responsibility for health, social support, and group work. It was founded as a non- profit organization.

3. *Self-Care for Senior Citizens, Hanover, NH*: The program uses an inter-disciplinary team approach to self-care education. It is affiliated with Dartmouth College Medical School.

4. *Senior Health Program of Augustana Hospital, Chicago, IL*: The program uses an interdisciplinary approach to patient education and activities. It is a permanent department of a religious hospital.

5. *The September Club, McLean, VA*: The club focuses on prevention, wellness, and social support; social workers are main staff persons. It is a proprietary enterprise.

6. *Health Aware, Toledo, OH*: The organization's purpose is adult education through groups on health promotion and disease prevention. It is a separate for-profit corporation of University of Toledo hospital.

(References for above programs: #1,2,3, and 4, in Health Promotion for Older Persons, 1982, #5 in Aptekar 1983, and #6 in Longe and Wolfe 1984.)

## Appendix B

Multiple Regression Analysis of Retirement, Death of a Spouse/ Significant Other, the Retirement x Income (T1) Interaction Plus the Control Variables as Predictors for Physical Health Satisfaction.

Least Squares Regression:　　　　　testing the *male* sample, N = 152

Outcome Variable: Phy Hlth Satis (T2)

| Predictor Variable | b | part r | beta |
|---|---|---|---|
| Retirement (T2) | -.85** | -.20 | -.44 |
| Death of a Spouse/Significant Other | .06 | .03 | .03 |
| Retirement x Income (T1) interaction | .14* | .16 | .38 |
| Controlling for: | | | |
| Prior Physical Health (T2) | .13*** | .26 | .26 |
| Age (T1) | .01 | .11 | .11 |
| Income (T1) | .03 | .04 | .07 |
| Income (T2) | .01 | .02 | .03 |
| Education (T1) | -.01 | -.06 | -.08 |
| Intercept | | 27.7 | |
| R | | .41 | |
| $R^2$ | | .17 | |
| F ratio | | 2.9*** | |

* $p<.10$; ** $p<.05$; *** $p<.01$

## Appendix C

Multiple Regression Analysis of Retirement, Death of a Spouse/ Significant Other, the Retirement x Death Interaction Plus the Control Variables as Predictors for Physical Health Satisfaction.


Least Squares Regression:          testing the *male* sample, N = 152

Outcome Variable: Phy Hlth Satis (T2)

| Predictor Variable | b | part r | beta |
|---|---|---|---|
| Retirement (T2) | -1.3* | -.17 | -.67 |
| Death of a Spouse/Significant Other | .06 | .03 | .03 |
| Retirment x Education interaction | .08 | .14 | .57 |
| Controlling for: | | | |
| Prior Physical Health (T2) | .13*** | .25 | .25 |
| Age (T1) | .01 | .09 | .09 |
| Income (T1) | .08 | .11 | .27 |
| Income (T2) | .01 | .02 | .03 |
| Education (T1) | -.03 | -.12 | -.14 |
| Intercept | | 24.7 | |
| R | | .40 | |
| $R^2$ | | .16 | |
| F ratio | | 2.8*** | |

* $p<.10$; ** $p<.05$; *** $p<.01$

# Appendix D

Multiple Regression Analysis of Retirement, the Retirement x Age Interaction Plus the Control Variables as Predictors for Physical Health Satisfaction.

Least Squares Regression: testing the *male* sample, N = 152

Outcome Variable: Phy Hlth Satis (T2)

| Predictor Variable | b | part r | beta |
|---|---|---|---|
| Retirement (T2) | -20.7 | -.04 | -10.7 |
| Retirement x Age interaction | -.01 | -.04 | -10.6 |
| Controlling for: | | | |
| Prior Physical Health (T2) | .14*** | .27 | .27 |
| Age (T1) | .01 | .11 | .13 |
| Income (T1) | .09 | .13 | .20 |
| Income (T2) | .008 | .011 | .02 |
| Education (T1) | -.01 | -.06 | -.07 |
| Intercept | | 32.2 | |
| R | | .38 | |
| R$^2$ | | .14 | |
| F ratio | | 2.8*** | |

* p<.10; ** p<.05; *** p<.01

## Appendix E

Multiple Regression Analysis of Retirement, Death of a Spouse/ Significant Other, the Retirement x Age Interaction Plus the Control Variables as Predictors for Physical Health Satisfaction.

Least Squares Regression:    testing the *male* sample, N = 152

Outcome Variable: Phy Hlth Satis (T2)

| Predictor Variable | b | part r | beta |
|---|---|---|---|
| Retirement (T2) | -22.05 | -.04 | -11.3 |
| Death of a Spouse/Significant Other | .04 | .02 | .01 |
| Retirement x Age interaction | -.01 | -.04 | -11.2 |
| Controlling for: | | | |
| Prior Physical Health (T2) | .14*** | .27 | .27 |
| Age (T1) | .01 | .11 | .13 |
| Income (T1) | .09 | .13 | .20 |
| Income (T2) | .009 | .01 | .02 |
| Education (T1) | -.01 | -.06 | -.07 |
| Intercept | | 33.08 | |
| R | | .38 | |
| $R^2$ | | .15 | |
| F ratio | | 2.5*** | |

\* p<.10; \*\* p<.05; \*\*\* p<.01

# BIBLIOGRAPHY

Adam, J. (1980). Stress and the risk of illness. In J. Adams (ed.), *Understanding and Managing Stress*, San Diego, CA: University Associates Inc.

Anderson, W.F. (1981). Is health education for the middle-aged and elderly a waste of time? *Family and Community Health*, 3,(4), 1-10.

Antonucci, T.C. (1983). Personal Characteristics, Social Support and Social Behavior. In E. Shanas and R.H. Binstock (eds.) *Handbook of Aging and the Social Sciences*, 2nd edition, NY:VanNostrand Co.

Antonucci, T.C. and House, J.S. (1983). Health and social support among the elderly. Institute for Social Research, University of Michigan.

Antonucci, T.C. and Jackson, J.S. (1983). Physical health and self-esteem. *Family & Community Health*, 1-9.

Apgar, K. and Coplon, J.K. (1985). New perspectives on structured life education groups, *Social Work*, 30,(2), 138-143.

Atchley, R.C. (1976). *The Sociology of Retirement*, Cambridge, MA: Schenkman Publishing Co.,Inc.

Atchley, R.C. (1982). Retirement as a social institution. *Ann. Rev. Sociol.*, 8, 263-287.

Barbaro, E.L. and Noyes, L.E. (1984). A wellness program for a life-care community. *The Gerontologist*, 24(6), 568-571.

Barney, J.L. and Neukom, J.E. (1977). Elderly users of health services. Institute of Gerontology, University of Michigan, Ann Arbor, MI.

Baur, P.A. and Okun, M.A. (1983). Stability of life satisfaction late life. *The Gerontologist*, 23(3), 261-265.

Birren, J.E. (1976) Psychological Aspects of Aging: intellectual functioning. In C.S. Kart and B.B. Manard, (eds.), *Aging in America*, Alfred Publishing Co.

Bloom, M. (1980). Primary prevention: revolution in the helping professions, *Social Work in Health Care*, 6(2), 53-67.

Bortz, E.L. (1972). Beyond retirement. In F. M. Carp (ed.), *Retirement*, New York: Behavioral Publications Inc., 339-366.

Bradford, L.P. (1979). Can you survive your retirement? *Harvard Business Review*, Nov-Dec, 103-109.

Branch, L.G., Katz, S., Kniepmann, K., and Papsidero, J.A. (1984). A prospective study of functional status among community elders, *American Journal of Public Health*, 74(3), 266-268.

Butler, R.N., Gertman, J.S., Oberlander, D.L. and Schindler, L. (1979). Self-care, self-help, and the elderly. *International Journal of Aging and Human Development*, 10(1), 95-117.

Cameron, K.A. and Persinger, M.A. (1983). Pensioners who die soon after retirement can be discriminated from survivors by post-retirement activities. *Psychological Reports*, 53, 564-66.

Campbell, A., Converse, P.E. and Rodgers, W.L. (1976). *The Quality of American Life: perceptions, evaluations, and satisfactions*. New York: Russell Sage Foundation.

Caspi, A. and Elder, G.H. (1986). Life satisfaction in old age: linking social psychology and history. *Journal of Psychology and Aging*, 1(1), 18-26.

Cassel, J. (1976a). The contribution of the social environment to host resistance, *American Journal of Epidemiology*, 104(2), 107-122.

Cassel, J. (1976b). Physical illness in response to stress. In S. Levine and N. Scotch (eds.), *Social Stress*, Aldine Publishing Co.

Checkoway, B.N. (1988). Community-based Initiatives to improve the Health of the Elderly. (to be published in the *Danish Medical Bulletin*).

Checkoway, B.N. and Betancourt, R.L. (1989). Community based initiatives to promote the health of the elderly in industrial and developing nations: lessons from the literature. (Paper submitted for publication).

Cluff, L.E. (1983). Problems of the health-impaired elderly: a foundations experience in geriatrics, *Journal of the American Geriatrics Society*, 31(11), 665-672.

Coyne, J.C. and DeLongis, A. (1986). Going beyond social support: the role of social relationships in adaptation. *Journal of Clinical and Consulting Psychology*, 54(4), 454-460.

Crump, C.E. and Lewis, C.B. (1985). Implications for the individual and the community. In C.B. Lewis (ed.), *Aging:the Health Care Challenge*, Philadelphia: F.A. Davis.

Cutrona, C., Russell, D., and Rose, J. (1986). Social support and adaptation to stress by the elderly. *Journal of Psychology and Aging*, 1(1), 47-54.

Dana, B. (1983). The social work-community medicine connection. *Social Work in Health Care*, 8(3), 11-23.

Durbin, N.E., Gross, E. and Borgatta, E.F. (1984). The decision to leave work. *Research on Aging*, 6, (4), 572-591.

Dychtwald, K. (1978). The Sage Project....a new image of age. *Journal of Humanistic Psychology*, 18(2), 69-74.

Dychtwald, K. (1983). Overview: health promotion and disease prevention for the elderly, *Generations*, VII(3), 5-7.

Eckstein, D. (1976). Common complaints of the elderly. *Hospital Practice*, (April), 67-74.

Eisdorfer, C. (1972). Adaptation to loss of work. In F.M. Carp (ed.), *Retirement*, NY:Behavioral Publications, 245-266.

Ekerdt, D.J., Baden, L., Bosse, R. and Dibbs, E. (1983). The effect of retirement on physical health. *American Journal of Public Health*, 73, (7), 779-783.

Elwell, F. and Maltbie-Crannell, A.D. (1981). The impact of role loss upon coping resources and life satisfaction of the elderly. *Journal of Gerontology*, 36(2), 223-232.

Fillenbaum, G.G. (1971). On the relation between attitude to work and attitude to retirement. *Journal of Gerontology*, 26, (2), 244-248.

Ford, A.B. (1981). Is health promotion affordable for the elderly? *Family and Community Health*, 3(4), 29-38.

German, P.S. (1975). Characteristics and health behavior of the aged population. *Gerontologist*, 8, 327-331.

Goudy, W. and Reger, R. (1985). Retirement attitudes and adjustment. In E. A. Powers, W. J. Goudy, P. M. Keith (eds.), *Later Life Transitions: Older Males in Rural America*, Boston: Kluwer-Nijhoff Publishers.

Green, K. (1985). Health promotion: its terminology, concepts, and modes of practice. *Health Values*, 9(3), 8-14.

Gurin, G., Veroff, J., and Feld, S. (1960). *Americans View their Mental Health*. New York: Basic Books.

Gustman, A.L. and Steinmeier, T.L. (1984). Partial retirement and the analysis of retirement behavior. *Industrial and Labor Relations Review*, 37(3), 403-410.

Guttman, D. (1978). Life events and decision-making by older adults. *The Gerontologist*, 18, (5), 462-467.

Hansson, R.O. (1986). Relational competence, relationships and adjustment in old age. *Personality and Social Psychology*, 50(5), 1050-1058.

Haynes, S.G., McMichael, A.J., and Tyroler, H.A. (1977). The relationship of normal involuntary retirement to early mortality among U.S. rubber workers. *Social Science and Medicine*, 11, 105-114.

*Health Care for Elders: alternative futures*. Select Committee on Aging, House of Representatives. Anaheim, CA, March 18, 1984.

*Health Maintenance and Health Promotion*. Report of the Technical Committee. The 1981 White House Conference on Aging, Washington, D.C.

*Health promotion for older persons: group program models*. Proceedings of the seminar: wellness--a community-based program approach. June 1982, National Council on Aging.

Heller, K., Swindle, R.W., and Dusenbury, L. (1986). Component social support processes: commments and integration. *Journal of Consulting and Clinical Psychology*, 54(4), 466-470.

Hetherington, R.W. and Calderone, G.E. (1985). Prevention and Health Policy: a view from the Social Sciences. *Public Health Reports*, 100(5), 507-514,

Hickey, T. (1980). *Health and Aging*. Monterey, CA: Brooks/Cole Publishers.

Holmes, T.H. and Rahe, R.H. (1967). The Social Readjustment Scale. *Journal of Psychosomatic Research*, 11, 213-218.

House, J. S., Robbins, C. and Metzner, H.L. (1982). The association of social relationships and activities with mortality: prospective evidence from the Tecumseh community health study. *American Journal of Epidemiology*, 116(1), 123-140.

Ingersoll, B.N. (1982). Gender differences in social support and quality of life among retirees. Unpublished doctoral dissertation, The University of Michigan.

Israel, B. (1988). Community-based social network interventions: meeting the needs of the elderly. (to be published in the *Danish Medical Bulletin*).

Jackson, J.S. and Gibson, R.C. (1983). Work and retirement among the black elderly. In Z. Blau (ed.), *Current Perspectives on Aging and the Life Cycle.*

Jacobs, B. and Abbott, S.D. (1983). Planning for wellness: a community-based approach. *Generations*, VII(3), 57-59.

Johnson, D.D. (1984). Medical self-care in the community. *Health Values*, 8(5), 13-14.

Kahn, R.L. and Antonucci, T.C. (1980). Social Networks in Adult Life. Survey Research Center, University of Michigan, Ann Arbor, MI.

Kahn, R.L. and Antonucci, T.C. (1984). Cancer Symptoms in the Elderly. Survey Research Center, University of Michigan, Ann Arbor, MI.

Keith, P.M. (1985). Work, retirement, and well-being among unmarried men and women. *The Gerontologist*, 25, (4), 410-416.

Kessler, R.C. (1982). Life events, social supports, and mental health. In Gove, W.R. (ed.), *Deviance and Mental Illness*, Beverly Hills, CA: Sage Press.

Krehl, W.A. (1983). The role of nutrition in maintaining health and preventing disease. *Health Values*, 7(2), 9-13.

Kremer, Y. (1985). The association between health and retirement: self-health assessment of Israeli retirees. *Social Science and Medicine*, 20(1), 61-66.

Lawton, M.P. and Brody, E. (1969). Assessments of older people: self-maintaining and instrumental activities of daily living. *Gerontologist*, 9, 179.

Lazarus, R.S. and DeLongis, A. (1983). Psychological stress and coping in aging. *American Psychologist*, March, 245-254.

Lederman, S., Rothschild, E., Farrar, M., and Spilka, L. (1983). The Wisdom Project: a community-based education program. *Generations*, VII(3), 48-49.

Levitt, M.J., Antonucci, T.C., Clark, M.C., Rotton, J., and Finley, G.E. (1982). Social support and well-being: preliminary indicators based on two samples of the elderly. *International Journal of Aging and Human Development.*

Lieberman, M.A. (1986). Social supports--the consequences of psychologizing: a commentary. *Journal of Consulting and Clinical Psychology*, 54(4), 461-465.

Lin, N., Simeone, R.S., Ensel, W.M., and Kuo, W. (1979). Social support, stressful life events, and illness: a model and an empirical test. *Journal of Health and Social Behavior*, 20, 108-119.

Linn, M.W. (1986). Modifiers and perceived stress scale. *Journal of Consulting and Clinical Psychology*, 54(4), 507-513.

Longe, M.E. and Wolf, A. (1984). *Promoting Community Health through Innovative Hospital-based Programs*. Chicago,IL: American Hospital Publishing Co.

Lorig, K., Laurin, J., and Holman, H.R. (1984). Arthritis self-Mmnagement: a study of the effectiveness of patient education for the elderly. *The Gerontologist*, 24(5), 455-457.

Love, J. W. (1980). Employment status after coronary bypass operations. *Journal of Thoracic and Cardiovascular Surgery*, 80, 68-72.

Lowenthal, M.F. (1964). *Lives in Distress*. New York: Basic Books.

Lurie, A. and Shulman, L. (1983). The professional connection with self-help groups in health care settings. *Social Work in Health Care*, 8(4), 69-77.

MacBride, A. (1976). Retirement as a life crisis: myth or reality? *Canadian Psychiatric Association Journal*, 21, 547-556.

Maddox, G.L. (1970). Adaptation to retirement. *The Gerontologist*, Spring, 14-18.

Maddox, G.L. and Douglass, E.B. (1973). Self-assessments of health: a longitudinal study of elderly subjects. *Journal of Health and Social Behavior*, 14, 87-93.

Mechanic, D. (1979). *Future Issues in Health Care*. New York: The Free Press.

Minkler, M. (1981). Applications of social support theory to health education: implications for work with the elderly. *Health Education Quarterly*, 8(2), 147-165.

Minkler, M. (1981). Research on the health effects of retirement: an uncertain legacy. *Journal of Health and Social Behavior*, 22, 117-130.

Minkler, M. (1988). Community-based initiatives to reduce isolation and enhance empowerment of the elderly: case studies from the United States. (to be published in the *Danish Medical Bulletin*).

Monnig, R. (1980). Self-care activities of older women. Paper presented at the November 1980 meeting of the Gerontological Society of America, San Diego, CA.

Morrison, M.H. (1983). The aging of the U.S. population: human resource implications. *Monthly Labor Review,* (May), 13-19.

Mutran, E. and Reitzes, D.C. (1981). Retirement, identity, and well-being: realignment of role relationships. *Journal of Gerontology*, 36(6), 733-740.

Nadelson, T. (1969). A survey of the literature on the adjustment of the aged to retirement. *Journal of Geriatric Psychiatry*,III, Fall 1, 3-19.

Nickoley-Colquitt, S. (1981). Preventive group interventions for elderly clients: are they effective? *Family and Community Health*, 3(4), 67-86.

Northen, H. (1983). Social work groups in health settings: promises and problems. *Social Work in Health Care,* 8(3), 107-121.

Palmore, E.B. (1964). Retirement patterns among aged men: findings of the 1963 survey of the aged. *Social Security Bulletin*, August, 3-10.

Palmore, E.B. (1976). The effects of aging on activities and attitudes. In Kart and Manard (eds.), *Aging in America*, Alfred Publishing Co.

Palmore, E.B., Cleveland, W.P., Nowlin, J.B., Ramm, D. and Siegler, I.C. (1979). Stress and adaptation in later life. *Journal of Gerontology*, 34(6), 841-851.

Palmore, E.B., Burchett, B.M., Fillenbaum, G.G., George, L.K. and Wallman, L.M. (1985). *Retirement: causes and consequences*. New York: Springer Publishing Co.

Parnes, H.S. and Nestel, G. (1981). The retirement experience. In H.S. Parnes (ed.), *Work and Retirement-a longitudinal study of men*, Cambridge, MA: The MIT Press.

Peck, T., VanVorst, J.R., and Root, J.A. (1983). *Wellness: the Revolution in Health Care*. St. Louis,MO: The Catholic Health Association of the United States.

Pelletier, K.R. (1983). Stress Management: an approach to optimum health and longevity. *Generations*, VII(3), 26-29.

Peppers, L.G. (1976). Patterns of leisure and adjustment to retirement. *The Gerontologist*, 16(5), 441-446.

Preston, D.B. and Mansfield, P.R. (1984). An exploration of stressful life events, illness, and coping among the rural elderly. *The Gerontologist*, 24(5), 490-494.

Quinn, J.F. (1981). The extent and correlates of partial retirement. *The Gerontologist*, 21(6), 634-643.

Rabin, D.L. (1984). Waxing of the gray, waning of the free. In *Health in an Older Society* by the Committee on an Aging Society, National Institute on Aging, Washington, D.C.

Rakowski, W. (1979). Future time perspective in later adulthood: review and research directions. *Experimental Aging Research*, 5(1), 43-48.

Rakowski, W. (1985). Preventive Health Behavior and Health Maintenance Practices of Older Adults. In B. Holstein, K. Dean, and T. Hickey (eds.), *Self-care and Health Behavior in Later Adulthood*, Croom-Helm, Ltd.

Roberto, K.A. and Scott, J.P. (1986). Friendships of older men and women: exchange patterns and satisfaction. *Psychology and Aging*, 1(2), 103-109.

Robinson, P.K., Coberly, S. and Paul, C.E. (1985). Work and Retirement. In R.H. Binstock and E. Shanas (eds.), *Handbook of Aging and the Social Sciences*, 2nd edition, New York: VanNostrand.

Rodgers, W.L. and Converse, P.E. (1975). Measures of the perceived overall quality of life. *Social Indicators Research*, 2, 127-152.

Russell, L.B. (1981). An aging population and the use of medical care. *Medical Care*, XIX(6), 633-643.

Ryff, C.D. (1986). Psychosocial well-being in adulthood and aging. American Psychological Association meeting, Washington, D.C., 1986.

Schaefer, C., Coyne, J.C., and Lazarus, R.S. (1981). The health-related functions of social support. *Journal of Behavioral Medicine*, 4(4), 381-405.

Schnore, M.M. (1985). *Retirement: Bane or Blessing?*, Waterloo, Canada: Wilfred Laurier University Press.

Schrock, M.M. (1980). *Holistic Assessment of the Healthy Aged.* New York: John Wiley & Sons.

Sells, S.B. (1970). On the nature of stress. In J.E. McGrath (ed.), *Social and Psychological Factors in Stress*. New York: Holt, Rinehart, and Winston, Inc.

Selye, H. (1974). *Stress without Distress*, London: Hodder and Stoughton.

Shamansky, S.L. and Hamilton, W.M. (1979). The Health Behavior Awareness Test: self-care education for the elderly. *Journal of Gerontological Nursing*, 5(1), 29-32.

Shanas, E. (1980). The Status of Health Care for the Elderly. In G. Lesnoff-Caravaglia (ed.), *Health Care of the Elderly*, New York: Human Services Press.

Shanas, E. and Maddox, G.L. (1983). Health, Health Resources, and the Utilization of Care. In Binstock and Shanas (eds.), *Handbook of Aging and the Social Sciences*, 2nd Edition, NY:VanNostrand.

Shannon, B.M., Smiciklas-Wright, H., Davis, B.W., and Lewis, C. (1983). A peer educator approach to nutrition for the elderly. *The Gerontologist*, 23(2), 123-126.

Siefert, K. (1983). An exemplar of primary prevention in social work: the Sheppard-Towner Act of 1921. *Social Work in Health Care*, 9(1), 87-103.

Simmons, J.J., Robert, E., and Nelson, E.C. (1983). Selfcare: tools, strategies and methods. *Generations*, VII(3), 46-47,64.

Sorenson, A.W. and Ford, M. (1981). Diet and health for senior citizens: workshops by the health team. *The Gerontologist*, 21(3), 257-262.

Spring, J. C. (1981). Medicare: an advocacy perspective for social workers. *Social Work in Health Care*, 6(4), 77-89.

Stokes, R.G. and Maddox, G.L. (1967). Some social factors on retirement adaptation. *Journal of Gerontology*, 22, 329-333.

Stults, B. (1984). Preventive Health Care for the Elderly. *Western Journal of Medicine*, 12(141), 832-845.

Tausig, M. (1986). Prior history of illness in the basic model. In Lin et al(eds.), *Social Support, Life Events and Depression*, Orlando, FL: Academic Press.

TenHoor, W.J. (1982). United States: Health and Personal Social Services. In M.C. Hokenstad and R.A. Ritvo, (eds.), *Linking Health Care and Social Services: International Perspectives*, Beverly Hills: Sage Publications.

Thoits, P.A. (1986). Social support as coping assistance. *Journal of Consulting and Clinical Psychology*, 54(4), 416-428.

Wallston, B.S., Alegna, S.W., DeVellis, S.M. and DeVellis, R.F., (1983). Social support and physical health, *Health Psychology*, 2(4), 367-382.

Wan, T.T.H., Odell, B.G., and Lewis, D.T. (1982). *Promoting the Well-Being of the Elderly: a community diagnosis.* New York: The Haworth Press.

Warner-Reitz, A. and Mettler, M.M. (1983). Designing health promotion programs for elders. *Generations*, VII, (3), 50-52, 66.

Wells, T. (1982). *Aging and Health Promotion.* Rockville, MD: Aspen Systems Publications.

Wethington, E. and Kessler, R.C. (1986). Perceived support, received support, and adjustment to stressful life events. *Journal of Health and Social Behavior*, 27, March, 78-89.

Whitbourne, S.K. and Sperneck, D.J. (1981). Health care and maintenance for the elderly. *Family and Community Health*, 3(4), 11-28.

Wolf, S. (1981). *Social Environment and Health,* Seattle: University of Washington Press.

Wolfe, B. and Wolfe, B. (1975). Exploring retirement in a small group. *Social Work*, November, 481-484.

World Health Organization, Regional Offices for Europe. The public health aspects of the aging of the population. Report of an advisory group, Oslo, July 28-August 2, 1958. Copenhagen: WHO, 1959.

Wylie, C.M. (1984). Contrasts in the health of elderly men and women, *Journal of the American Geriatrics Society*, September, 32(9), 670-675.